The Demand for Military Health Care

Supporting Research for a Comprehensive Study of the Military Health-Care System

*Susan D. Hosek, Bruce W. Bennett,
Joan L. Buchanan, M. Susan Marquis,
Kimberly A. McGuigan, Janet M. Hanley,
Rodger Madison, Afshin Rastegar,
Jennifer Hawes-Dawson*

*Prepared for the
Office of the Secretary of Defense*

National Defense Research Institute

Preface

This report documents supporting research for the Comprehensive Study of the Military Medical Care System, which was requested by the National Defense Authorization Act for Fiscal Years 1992 and 1993. Within the Department of Defense, the study was entrusted to the Director of Program Analysis and Evaluation (PA&E), who asked RAND to undertake research on the utilization of health care by military beneficiaries and the costs of care provided through the Civilian Health and Medical Program of the Uniformed Services (CHAMPUS). The analyses cover current utilization and costs, and they project utilization and costs for several analytic cases that alter the structure of the military system. In its report to Congress, PA&E assessed the total costs of the military system by combining the results of this research with research conducted by the Institute for Defense Analyses on the costs of care provided in military health facilities.

The work reported here was sponsored by PA&E and was carried out within the Forces and Resources Policy Center of RAND's National Defense Research Institute (NDRI). NDRI is a federally funded research and development center sponsored by the Office of the Secretary of Defense, the Joint Staff, and the defense agencies.

Contents

Figures

Tables

Summary

The Military Health Services System (MHSS) provides health care to active-duty service members, military retirees, and their dependents. Over the past several years, the system has faced the twin challenges of downsizing in consonance with the rest of the Department of Defense (DoD) and of controlling escalating health care costs. These challenges cannot, however, be dealt with independently. Closing military treatment facilities (MTFs) could drive non-active-duty beneficiaries to seek more expensive medical care from the civilian sector, care that is reimbursed by DoD through the Civilian Health and Medical Program of the Uniformed Services (CHAMPUS). In 1991, in response to a congressional request, the Director of Program Analysis and Evaluation (PA&E) undertook an evaluation of health care utilization and costs within the current system and of various possible alternatives to that system. PA&E turned to RAND's National Defense Research Institute (NDRI) for analytic support in responding to Congress. Specifically, we were asked to compare current utilization by military beneficiaries with use by civilians, to develop analytic cases to study alternatives to the current medical structure, and to assess costs and changes in utilization associated with these cases (with the exception of MTF costs, which are being assessed by the Institute for Defense Analyses).

We compared utilization data from a survey fielded as part of the PA&E study with data from ongoing civilian-sector surveys. After correcting for demographic differences and other factors unrelated to military service that might influence health care use, we were able to verify previous research findings that utilization by military beneficiaries is higher than use in the civilian sector. We found that the rates at which military beneficiaries used inpatient and outpatient services were on the order of 30 to 50 percent higher than those of civilians in fee-for-service plans. We suspect that these differences result from the more generous health benefits available in the military, from the greater risk of injury faced by service members in contrast to civilians, from military practice patterns and work-excuse rules, and from the influence of those factors on the proclivity of military families to use health care services.

Surveys are not the only source of data on utilization by military beneficiaries. The MHSS collects its own data, data that suggest dramatically different utilization rates for some groups of beneficiaries. After careful review, we found that various aspects of MHSS data collection, recording, and reporting can make it difficult to draw reliable inferences from these data on health care utilization. These findings suggest that caution be exercised in the uncritical use of such data.

We developed analytic cases that incorporate four very different ways of providing military health care in the future. The first two cases stipulate modified versions of the current MHSS:

- Nationwide implementation of managed-care options such as those now in place in California, Hawaii, the Southeast, and elsewhere. DoD has now amassed considerable experience with these options and expects that with some modifications, they will control costs while improving beneficiary satisfaction.

- Expansion of the number of MTFs as well as the size and staffing of selected facilities. This alternative takes the system in the opposite direction from the current downsizing trend in the interests of shifting more dependents and retirees from CHAMPUS coverage to MTFs, which are generally thought to be less costly. It raises the question, however, as to whether increasing access to MTFs, where care is free to beneficiaries, might increase the demand for health care and draw in beneficiaries now using private health insurance plans.

In the other two cases, most beneficiaries would choose among several health plans. Both cases would offer commercial health plans; the first would close most MTFs and offer commercial plans only, whereas the second would retain the MTFs and allow beneficiaries who live near an MTF to choose between an MTF-based plan and commercial plans.

- Reduce the number of military hospitals from more than 100 to around 10, enough to handle casualties returning from an overseas conflict either through treatment or through referral to civilian-sector hospitals. Under this alternative, most hospitals at military installations would survive only as outpatient clinics. All non-active-duty beneficiaries would enroll in civilian managed-care health plans, and care for active-duty personnel beyond what the clinics could provide would be furnished by civilian-sector providers under the supervision of the clinics. This alternative would greatly reduce MTF fixed costs while putting into place a mechanism for controlling civilian-sector costs.

- Establish competing military and civilian health care plans: one health maintenance organization (HMO) operated by military hospitals and the others by commercial plans. Service members would enroll in the military plan, while other beneficiaries would choose from among the military HMO and civilian plans. This would allow DoD to take advantage of the usual efficiency enhancements that result from competition.

For the first two analytic cases, our analysis was based on what we know about the way in which utilization by military beneficiaries currently rests on the cost and availability of military and civilian health care resources. We projected that MTF utilization in the expanded-MTF case would be roughly 15 percent greater than that in the modified current system envisioned in the first case but that CHAMPUS-funded use would be less, albeit not by as much—only by enough to permit a 9 percent drop in CHAMPUS costs. For every CHAMPUS visit not made in the expanded-MTF case, 1.7 additional visits would be made at the MTF; for every CHAMPUS hospitalization avoided, 3.4 additional patients are admitted to the MTF.

Cases 3 and 4 envision more far-reaching changes in the MHSS and so our analysis also incorporated information about health care utilization and costs in the civilian sector. Using hypothetical health-plan choices reported in the beneficiary survey, we concluded that between 60 and 70 percent of military families would prefer a civilian health plan to a military health plan if the two plans covered the same services and required the same cost sharing. However, if the family would have to pay a premium contribution for the civilian plan, but not for the military plan, most families would prefer the military plan. To induce enough families (65–70 percent) to choose the military plan to sustain the current MTF system, we estimate that DoD would have to charge $50 per month per family for civilian plans. CHAMPUS-eligible families are more sensitive to premium contribution levels than Medicare-eligible families.

Civilian plan costs varied only slightly by case and type of plan—fee-for-service (FFS) or health maintenance organization (HMO). We predicted costs for FFS plans from a simulation model of health care expenditures, based on the benefit package currently provided by CHAMPUS. *For those families we predicted would choose a civilian FFS plan*, we estimated FY92 per-person costs of approximately $2,100 for dependents of junior enlisted personnel, $1,950 for other active-duty dependents, and $2,900 for retirees and their dependents. Out-of-pocket costs range from $200 for active-duty dependents to over $600 for retirees and dependents. These estimates assume enrolled beneficiaries receive all their health care through this FFS plan. We determined HMO costs from the premiums charged by HMOs participating in the Federal Employees Health Benefits Program; in FY92, these HMOs charged $1,850 for a single person and $4,625 for a family. Although individual HMOs charge more or less than these amounts, we found little systematic variation in premiums across the country.

Case 4 envisions transforming the MTFs into a military HMO, responsible for providing all the health care for enrolled beneficiaries either directly or by purchasing civilian health care at MTF expense. Under this arrangement, the MTFs would have strong incentives to lower utilization. To determine the potential for lower MTF utilization in case 4, we estimated three sets of utilization for those families predicted to enroll in the MTF plan. The first set assumed that beneficiaries would continue to use health care at rates currently observed in areas with substantial MTF capacity. The second set assumed that utilization rates would decline to the rates we measured for comparable civilian HMO enrollees. The third set assumed that the MTFs would induce beneficiaries to use less care by charging a clinic fee. To reach HMO utilization levels, this fee would have to be equivalent to 25 percent of the average cost of a visit (perhaps $25). In general, we conclude that utilization could decline by 25 percent if the MTFs were restructured as an HMO.

Finally, we estimated the potential savings to DoD if the civilian employers of military beneficiaries were mandated to contribute 80 percent of the cost of the beneficiaries' health insurance and health reform were implemented in a manner that discouraged retaining dual coverage by employer plans and the MHSS. These savings would amount to $5 billion in 1994 dollars.

1. Introduction

Section 733 of the National Defense Authorization Act for Fiscal Years 1992 and 1993 requires that the Secretary of Defense conduct a comprehensive study of the military health care system to include two major elements: (1) a "systematic review of the . . . system required to support the Armed Forces during a war or other conflict and any adjustments to that system that would be required to provide cost-effective health care in peacetime"; and (2) a "comprehensive review of the existing . . . civilian health care . . . programs that are available as alternatives to . . . the existing military medical care system." Within the Department of Defense (DoD), this study was entrusted to the Director of Program Evaluation and Analysis (PA&E), who requested that RAND carry out supporting research on the peacetime demand for health care by military beneficiaries. The purpose of the current report is to document the first phase of this research. A subsequent version of the report will incorporate the rest of the research.

The congressional language also delineated some requirements for the content of the study report. With respect to the provision of peacetime health care, the report was to include:

- An evaluation of beneficiaries' utilization of inpatient and outpatient services, identifying deviations from utilization patterns in civilian health plans;

- A list of methods for providing care that are available as alternatives to the current military health care system;

- The relationship between the demand for health care and the availability of military medical resources;

- The likely response of beneficiaries to any planned changes in the costs they bear for care; and

- A comparison of the costs of providing care in military treatment facilities with those of indemnity plans or health maintenance organizations (HMOs).

We take up these items in order, following a brief description of the military health care system and of recent efforts to reform that system (Section 2). Section 3 then compares health service utilization in the military system with that of civilian health plans, investigates potential reasons for the differences measured, and compares measures of military utilization derived from different data sources. Section 4 describes in some detail the alternative systems that were developed as analytic cases for the study. Although the general shape of these cases was determined by PA&E, the details needed for analysis were developed by RAND. Estimates of the effects of two cases on health care utilization and civilian care costs are provided in Section 5; the effects of the other cases are discussed in Section 6.[1] We did not estimate the costs associated with utilization of military health facilities. This task was carried out by the Institute for Defense Analyses (IDA), based on utilization estimates we provided to them. The report concludes in Section 7 with some observations about the results.

This study of the military health care system was carried out as the nation considered health care reform. Even without federal legislation, the health care marketplace is undergoing extensive changes. The legislation submitted in the fall of 1993 by the President would have authorized DoD to establish one or more health plans and collect premium contributions from private employers of military beneficiaries who enroll in a military plan. DoD would have had wide latitude in structuring its health program, so any of the alternatives developed as analytic cases for this study could be pursued with national health reform. However, with or without federal action, national reform will alter DoD's health care costs and may affect beneficiaries' use of the military system under all alternatives. An analysis of the potential impact of national reform was beyond the scope of this study, but we did roughly estimate the savings DoD might realize if private employers were required to offer their employees health care benefits.

---

[1]We did not analyze the effects of alternative systems on other health care outcomes, such as patient satisfaction or health status. These outcomes are addressed elsewhere in the study.

2. Structure of the Current Military Health Services System

The Military Health Services System (MHSS) provides health care to roughly 9.2 million beneficiaries, including active-duty military personnel and their dependents, retired military personnel and their dependents, and survivors of military personnel.[1] Approximately 8.5 million of these beneficiaries live in the United States, where at the end of FY92 the MHSS provided direct military care through 117 military hospitals and some 400 military clinics.[2] With military downsizing and base closures, the number of military facilities has declined and is expected to continue to decline such that by about 1997 only 101 military hospitals are expected to remain in operation.[3] The MHSS augments this military treatment facility (MTF) system with CHAMPUS,[4] a health insurance plan that finances civilian health care for most non-active-duty beneficiaries under the age of 65. Since MTF care is free, whereas CHAMPUS requires beneficiary cost sharing, the real benefits available to military beneficiaries are greater for those living near an MTF.

Health Care Services in Military Treatment Facilities

Military hospitals provide care to all military beneficiaries free of charge as capacity permits. By law, such hospitals accord first priority to active-duty personnel, followed by active-duty dependents and then retirees, their dependents, and other beneficiaries (see Figure 1).

These hospitals vary widely both in size and in the range of services they can provide. The largest are medical centers, which have hundreds of operating beds each and which offer a comprehensive range of health care services; medical centers also provide graduate medical education (GME) to train many of the

---

[1]In addition, the MHSS provides health care for National Guard and Reserve members serving on active duty (and their families), civilian employees at selected DoD facilities, and other beneficiaries of government health care.

[2]The almost 400 military clinics mentioned here independently report workload and other data into biometrics military data systems; other clinics report data only through their parent hospitals. We have not included Coast Guard clinics or U.S. treatment facilities (formerly the Public Health Service hospitals).

[3]This assumes that all planned base closures are ultimately implemented, including those in the 1993 BRAC (Base Realignment and Closing) actions.

[4]Civilian Health and Medical Program of the Uniformed Services.

4

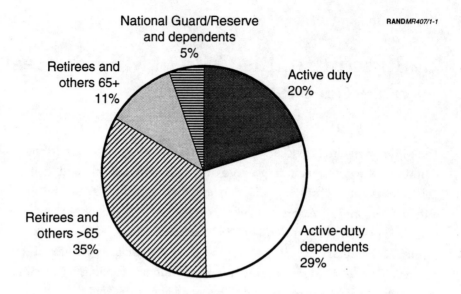

RAND*MR407/1-1*

National Guard/Reserve
and dependents
5%

Retirees and
others 65+
11%

Active duty
20%

Retirees and
others >65
35%

Active-duty
dependents
29%

Figure 1—Composition of the Military Beneficiary Population, FY92

doctors who will be used by the military. The remaining hospitals can be classified either as small hospitals—those that operate fewer than 70 beds and provide basic medical care—or as medium hospitals that operate from 70 to about 200 beds and offer a broader range of services, albeit not as broad as those of medical centers. At the end of 1992, the MHSS had 69 small hospitals, 30 medium hospitals, and 18 medical centers; by 1997, the MHSS will have 60 small hospitals, 24 medium hospitals, and 17 medical centers.

Each military hospital has a defined service area—called a catchment area. This area generally includes the zip code areas within 40 miles of the hospital. Maps of the continental United States, showing the location of the MTFs still open in 1997, may be found at the end of Section 4. Many MTFs are located in the Southeast and Southwest. Most military beneficiaries live near an MTF. Military hospitals and their associated outpatient clinics serve 87 percent of all active-duty personnel, 80 percent of their dependents, and 57 percent of retirees and all other beneficiaries. Including freestanding military clinics, these percentages rise to 90, 89, and 68, respectively.

A few catchment areas have extended their MTF capacity through PRIMUS/NAVCARE clinics. These clinics, which are operated by civilian contractors off-base, provide primary care at no cost to non-active-duty beneficiaries.

Some military bases have only a military outpatient clinic. Such military clinics provide care primarily to active-duty personnel; some provide little or no care to other beneficiaries, whereas others offer primary care and referrals as required to military or civilian specialists and hospitals. Some of the larger of these clinics also provide a "holding area"—an infirmary-like facility in which overnight care and observation can be provided, especially for active-duty personnel.

Outside of military hospitals and clinics, the military has a large number of corpsmen and doctors who serve as part of military units. For example, some doctors are assigned to ships, providing care for ship personnel both in port and while away from port. Finally, when necessary, the military also deploys "detached" medical facilities in the form of field hospitals and hospital ships. These facilities provide inpatient as well as outpatient services.

CHAMPUS

Non-active-duty beneficiaries under the age of 65 may also obtain health care from civilian providers through CHAMPUS. Beneficiaries living near an MTF, however, must use that MTF instead of CHAMPUS for high-cost outpatient services as well as for all inpatient services if such services are available there. This rule applies to all CHAMPUS-eligible beneficiaries who live in a given MTF's defined catchment area, which extends approximately 40 miles from that MTF. When military beneficiaries reach the age of 65, CHAMPUS eligibility automatically ends and Medicare coverage begins; eligibility for treatment at military facilities continues.

Under the standard CHAMPUS plan, beneficiaries who use a civilian provider for outpatient care face a small deductible along with a copayment of 20 to 25 percent. Active-duty dependents pay only a nominal copayment for civilian inpatient care, but retirees and dependents face the same copayment and deductible as those associated with outpatient care. The first column in Table 1 lists standard CHAMPUS benefits in more detail.

Ongoing Reform in the MHSS

Since 1988, DoD has experimented with several new programs that offer beneficiaries managed-care alternatives to the standard CHAMPUS plan with more generous benefits. Programs that were in operation at the end of 1992 included the CHAMPUS Reform Initiative (CRI), which is offered in California

Table 1

Benefits and Coverage of Various MHSS Plans, FY 1992

Benefit/ Coverage Element	Standard MTF/ CHAMPUS Plan	CRI/CAM Enrollment Plans	PPOs
Enrollment Fee	None	None	None
Military Treatment Facility Care			
Copayment	None	None	None
Services for which MTF may be required	Inpatient care; some high-cost outpatient services	All outpatient specialty and inpatient care	Inpatient care; some high-cost outpatient services
Civilian Care			
Annual deductible	Deps. of jr. enlisted: $50 individual, $100 family Others: $150 individual, $300 family	None in CRI, AF CAM 50% of standard deductible in Navy CAM	Same as standard deductible
Physician services copayment	Active-duty deps.: 20% of CHAMPUS allowable Others: 25% of CHAMPUS allowable	CRI: $5 per visit AF CAM: free primary care; standard copayment minus 5% otherwise Navy CAM: standard copayment minus 5%	Standard copayment minus 5%
Outpatient mental health copayment	Same as physician services copayment	CRI: $10 per individual visit; $5 per group visit CAM: Same	Same as standard deductible
Coverage for preventive services	No coverage except well-baby care and routine eye exams	Routine physical exams, Pap smears, and similar preventive care	Same as standard coverage
Hospitalization copayment			
Active-duty dependents	Greater of $25 or $8.05/day	No copayment	No copayment
Retired and dependents	Lesser of $175/day or 25% of charges	$75/day to $750 max. per admission	Lesser of $125/day or 25% of charges
Outpatient prescription copayment	Same as physician services copayment	CRI: $4 copayment CAM: Same	Same as standard copayment
Providers covered	Free to use any provider except if MTF is required	Must use network providers while enrolled	Must use network providers for episode of care
Paperwork required	Beneficiary often files own claim	No beneficiary claims filing	No beneficiary claims filing

and Hawaii;[5] the Catchment Area Management (CAM) program, which subsumes three catchment areas;[6] and a preferred-provider organization (PPO) in the Southeast. CRI and CAM were also designed to encourage better coordination between the MTFs and CHAMPUS, to improve beneficiary access and satisfaction, and to make the system more cost-effective. Specifically, CRI offers beneficiaries the choice of (1) remaining in the standard MTF/CHAMPUS plan, which is enhanced with an optional PPO that lowers the CHAMPUS copayment for beneficiaries who use selected civilian providers, or (2) enrolling in an HMO that eliminates most cost sharing for civilian care but covers only care that is obtained from MTFs or from selected civilian providers. The CAM programs offer beneficiaries a choice of either the standard plan (without the PPO option) or an HMO plan (Air Force) and a PPO plan (Navy).[7] Table 1 also summarizes the benefits offered in the CRI and CAM enrollment plans as well as in the optional PPO available both in the CRI and in the Southeast-region program.

On the basis of its experience with these programs, DoD has developed a permanent managed-care reform to the MHSS that is based on the CRI but encompasses some revision in its cost-sharing provisions. Most beneficiaries who enroll in the HMO option will pay a small annual enrollment fee and somewhat higher copayments for outpatient visits than they did in the early CRI programs. This reform is discussed further in Section 4. A related reform—capitation budgeting—will allocate health care resources to catchment areas on a per-capita basis. This reform is just now being implemented.

A key characteristic of the MHSS lies in its blending of military and civilian health care options in a single health plan, for which all military beneficiaries are automatically eligible (the reform programs offer additional choices).[8] Although some of the analytic cases considered in this study maintain the current structure, others involve more radical changes.

---

[5]For an evaluation of CRI, see Hosek et al. (1993) and Sloss and Hosek (1993). A similar evaluation of CAM is under way.

[6]The CAM demonstration program was implemented at five sites, but two of these sites were no longer operational by the end of 1992 because their demonstration authority had ended.

[7]The Army CAM program ended in FY92; its enrollment plan was an HMO.

[8]Enrollment is simple and occurs automatically as part of routine personnel processing, so almost all eligible beneficiaries are enrolled.

3. Health Care Utilization in the MHSS

Policymakers in DoD and Congress often ask whether military beneficiaries are underserved or overserved by the MHSS. Answering this question demands an assessment not just of the number of services beneficiaries use but also of the appropriateness and quality of the care provided. Nonetheless, utilization levels are broadly suggestive of the level of service available. Earlier studies of the military health care system found that utilization rates were substantially higher in the military than in the civilian population (Phelps et al., 1984; Congressional Budget Office, 1988); active-duty personnel appeared to make two to three times as many outpatient visits as did their civilian counterparts, in part because of the requirement for an unusually high state of health in the active-duty force. Active-duty dependents' utilization rates were also estimated to be 40 to 50 percent higher than those of the civilian population. Measured rates of retirees and their dependents were sometimes lower, but these rates did not account for all their use of health care services; the MHSS data used in the comparisons excluded utilization outside the military system. As part of the legislation mandating this study, Congress requested that a new comparison be made of military and civilian health care utilization. In this section, we present that comparison and explain the differences we found. We also show the sources of care used by military beneficiaries.

To compare military and civilian utilization rates, we used the beneficiary survey Congress included in its request for this study along with a national survey of the civilian population. To measure military utilization by source of care, we used the beneficiary survey together with routinely collected MHSS data. For various reasons, we found that these two data sources are not always comparable. Although greatly improved in recent years, MHSS data are prone to errors that limit their usefulness for calculating utilization rates, especially by geographic area. Because these limitations are likely to pose difficulties for many kinds of analyses, we devote some space to them in the second half of this section.

Military-Civilian Comparison

We compared two measures of annual health care use: the average number of outpatient visits per person and the percentage of recipients who had received any hospital care. Calculations of these measures were adjusted for differences in military and civilian populations in age, sex, and other characteristics known to affect utilization. We present comparisons for outpatient and inpatient use followed by some possible explanations for the differences we found. First, though, we review critical aspects of the surveys and comparison methodology.

Overall, this analysis tends to confirm the findings of earlier studies. Our results can be summarized as follows:

- Military beneficiaries use more health care than do comparable civilians. Much of this difference in utilization can be explained by the generosity of military health benefits, particularly the availability of free MTF care— although other factors may also come into play.

- Those beneficiaries with the highest priority for MTF care—active-duty personnel, followed by their dependents—obtain a large proportion of their care from MTFs and very little of that care from non-MHSS sources.

- Other beneficiaries—retirees, survivors, and their dependents—get less than half their care from MTFs if they live in catchment areas and almost none if they live in noncatchment areas. For those under age 65, CHAMPUS financed (at least in part) almost three-quarters of civilian outpatient care but only half as much civilian inpatient care. We should note, however, that these estimates are imprecise in that they rest on a comparison of CHAMPUS and survey data.

- Although MHSS data can generate reasonably accurate aggregate inpatient utilization rates for active-duty personnel and their dependents, the rates estimated by geographic location are unreliable. These data are similarly useful for measuring aggregate utilization of MHSS inpatient services for other beneficiaries, but they cannot be used to estimate total utilization.

- MHSS data yield substantially higher MTF outpatient utilization rates than do the beneficiary survey data. The reasons for this discrepancy, which is even larger when rates are calculated for specific geographic areas, cannot be investigated with current MHSS outpatient data systems. Therefore, MHSS outpatient data should be used with caution.

Overview of the Surveys Used in the Comparison

Data for civilian utilization rates were derived from the National Health Interview Survey (NHIS), which is fielded annually by the federal government to a sample of the U.S. civilian noninstitutionalized population.[1] The NHIS assesses health status and health service utilization by interviewing a sample of approximately 50,000 households and 120,000 individuals each year. We used the 1989 NHIS because that year's data contained information regarding insurance coverage—information that is essential to ensuring the comparability of the samples. To determine whether the different time periods for the two surveys would affect the comparison, we reviewed NHIS data for the years 1987 to 1991 for evidence of a trend in utilization. We found that outpatient use by the civilian population (e.g., visits per person) had not changed during these years and that inpatient admission rates had also remained constant, while the average length of a hospital stay had declined. By comparing the percentage of recipients hospitalized but not the number of hospital days, we thus concluded that we could use the 1989 NHIS.

To facilitate comparison, the questionnaire for this study's military beneficiary survey included the same questions on utilization and health status as those in the NHIS. The military survey was fielded by mail in late 1992 and early 1993 to a sample of 45,000 military households, whose sponsors were active-duty personnel with and without dependents, active and reserve retirees, and survivors of military personnel. We principally used the results from the portion of the survey that was directed toward one randomly selected member of each family. This portion asked for the number of outpatient visits, the number of hospital days (which we used to determine whether the person was hospitalized), and other information about this individual.

The sample for the military survey was randomly selected within each of 73 population strata, with different sampling rates used for the different strata.[2] To obtain estimates for the military population rather than just the survey sample, we weighted the survey data to account for different sampling and nonresponse rates. The methods we used to obtain survey weights are detailed in Appendix A.

Methods for Estimating Utilization Levels

We estimated utilization rates using NHIS and military survey data for individuals age 1 to 64 who lived in the United States. In the case of the NHIS, we excluded individuals without private-insurance coverage in efforts to render

---

[1]See the National Center for Health Statistics (1990) for a description of the 1989 survey.

[2]The strata were defined by beneficiary category (e.g., active duty, retired), family status (with or without dependents), and military health program type (e.g., CRI, Army CAM, noncatchment area).

the civilian sample more comparable to the military sample, all of whose members have health insurance. We excluded from the military sample survivor and retired Reserve/National Guard households as well as active-duty personnel who were considered to be afloat (but not their families). We then used standard regression analysis techniques to express health care utilization as a function of whether an individual belonged to the military or civilian population and of other characteristics potentially related to utilization: education, income, family size, and self-reported health status. We also included information on whether the individual was covered by a fee-for-service (FFS) or an HMO plan (for civilians) to permit estimates to be made for these different types of civilian health plans. Using the regression results, we then estimated average utilization levels for military beneficiaries and for comparable individuals in the civilian population. These estimates are thus adjusted for any military-civilian utilization differences other than whether or not an individual was a military beneficiary. Appendix B describes our methods in greater detail and reports the results of the regression analysis.

We compare utilization for five beneficiary groups: active-duty personnel, active-duty dependents, retirees under age 65, retirees' dependents under age 65, and retirees and dependents 65 and over. We report separate civilian utilization rates for HMOs and FFS plans for all the under-65 groups, as research has typically shown that HMOs experience higher outpatient utilization and lower inpatient utilization than do FFS plans. Since HMO enrollment rates are very low in the Medicare popualation, we do not report civilian rates by type of plan.

As a check on the comparability of these two surveys, we also compared utilization rates in the NHIS for civilians and the limited number of military beneficiaries included in the NHIS sample. In doing so, we were able to identify active-duty dependents but not military retirees. A comparison of utilization rates adjusted for age and sex (but not for health status) yielded results that were similar to those we obtained from comparing the military survey with the NHIS.

Comparison of Military and Civilian Outpatient Use

The first three columns of data in Table 2 show the average number of visits for each group of military beneficiaries and their counterparts in civilian FFS and HMO plans. For military beneficiaries, we include all visits, not just those made at MTFs or through CHAMPUS. As in earlier studies, we find that active-duty personnel and their dependents have substantially higher outpatient utilization levels. Compared with civilians in FFS plans, these differences—43 percent for active-duty personnel and 38 percent for dependents—are somewhat smaller

Table 2

Comparison of Outpatient Utilization in the Military Population and Comparable Civilian Populations

Beneficiary Group	Average Visits per Person			Probability of Having Any Visits		
		Civilian			Civilian	
	Military	FFS	HMO	Military	FFS	HMO
Active-duty personnel	3.09	2.16	2.28	0.82	0.68	0.70
Active-duty dependents	3.84	2.78	2.92	0.89	0.78	0.80
Retirees under 65	4.37	3.32	3.49	0.84	0.73	0.76
Retired dependents under 65	4.33	3.27	3.42	0.90	0.81	0.83
Retirees & dependents over 65	5.70	4.51[a]		0.91	0.91[a]	

NOTE: Estimates control for differences in sociodemographic characteristics and health status between the military and civilian populations. For all beneficiary groups, the differences in average visits between the military beneficiaries and both civilian groups are statistically significant at $p < .05$.

[a]Total for all-civilian.

than those previously measured. Outpatient utilization tends to be higher in HMOs than in FFS plans because the out-of-pocket cost is lower. Therefore, compared with civilian HMO enrollees, active-duty personnel and dependents make only 36 and 32 percent more visits, respectively.

When we consider all sources of care and not just MHSS sources, military retirees and their dependents under age 65 are also found to have higher visit rates, but the differences are about five percentage points lower than those for active-duty dependents. The difference is even smaller (26 percent) for beneficiaries 65 and over, almost all of whom get some care whether or not they are in the military population.

Military outpatient utilization rates may be underestimated somewhat in relation to civilian rates. The military survey windsorized the data at 10 visits—i.e., limited the number of visits that could be recorded for each health care location to 10 or more. We similarly limited the NHIS data. To the extent that the tendency for military beneficiaries to use more health care extends to those making more than 10 visits per year, we have underestimated military-civilian differences in utilization.[3]

---

[3]We considered correcting the military survey data instead of windsorizing the NHIS data. There are no similar data on military beneficiaries' self-reported utilization by source of care from which we could determine the frequency of visits above 10. Therefore, making this correction would have required that some assumptions be made about this frequency, which would have led to

The last three columns of data in Table 2 show the fraction of beneficiaries with any outpatient visits in comparable military and civilian populations. Generally, about one-third to one-half of the military-civilian differential is due to a higher probability of having any outpatient use at all. The remainder is attributable to an increased number of visits for those with some use.

Utilization rates are often reported by age and sex without adjusting for other health-related characteristics. Figures 2 and 3 compare outpatient visit rates by age and sex in the military survey with those in the MHIS. The age-sex utilization profiles for the two populations generally have the same shape. With the exception of the youngest children, however, military beneficiaries of both sexes average a higher number of outpatient visits at all ages.

Comparison of Military and Civilian Inpatient Use

All four military beneficiary groups also tend to display higher inpatient utilization rates, as measured by the annual probability of being hospitalized, than do persons who are similar but unconnected with the military (Table 3). Within the civilian population, the rate of hospitalization is usually found to be lower in HMOs than in FFS plans—a pattern we also find here.[4] Focusing on those in FFS plans, we see that the differential in military inpatient use is about equal to the outpatient differential for active-duty dependents and Medicare eligibles, but is smaller for the other beneficiary groups. The military differential is considerably higher if the civilian comparison group consists of HMO enrollees.

Why Do Military Beneficiaries Use More Health Care?

One explanation usually advanced for the higher health care use found in the military population pivots on the availability of free MTF care. Typical civilian health plans include a deductible, often in the amount of about $200 per individual, as well as a copayment of 20 percent. CHAMPUS has similar cost-sharing provisions, but, as shown below, MTFs provide roughly two-thirds of the care used by active-duty dependents and one-third of the care used by retirees and dependents. The differences we estimate—military utilization that is 32 to 43 percent higher than FFS outpatient use and 23 to 33 percent higher than

---

unknown biases in the estimates. We chose instead to windsorize the NHIS data because this approach would yield a conservative estimate of military-civilian utilization differences.

[4]See, for example, Bradbury et al. (1991), Luft (1981), Manning et al. (1984), and Welch (1985).

14

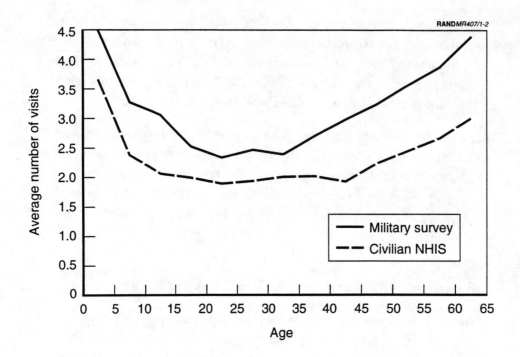

Figure 2—Average Self-Reported Outpatient Visits by Age and Sex, Males
(windsorized at 10 visits)

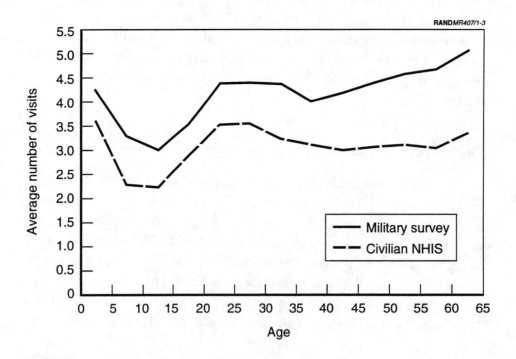

Figure 3—Average Self-Reported Outpatient Visits by Age and Sex, Females (excludes
active duty) (windsorized at 10 visits)

Table 3

**Comparison of Inpatient Utilization
in the Military Population and Comparable Civilian Populations**

| Beneficiary Group | Probability of Having Any Overnight Hospital Care | | |
| | Military | Civilian | |
		FFS	HMO
Active-duty personnel	0.095	0.073	0.065
Active-duty dependents	0.113	0.086	0.076
Retirees under 65	0.151	0.122	0.109
Retirees' dependents under 65	0.112	0.091	0.081
Retirees & dependents over 65	0.24	0.18	

NOTE: Estimates control for differences in sociodemographic characteristics and health status between the military and civilian populations. For all beneficiary groups, the differences in average visits between the military beneficiaries and both civilian groups are statistically significant at $p < .05$.

FFS inpatient use—are generally consistent with evidence on the effects of cost sharing.

The best evidence on the effects of cost sharing can be found in a large health-insurance experiment conducted in the 1970s. By randomly assigning families to insurance plans that differed only in their cost-sharing arrangements, the experiment estimated changes in the number of episodes of health care used due to cost sharing. Families assigned to a free plan had 41 percent more outpatient episodes than did families assigned to a plan with cost sharing and 21 percent more inpatient episodes (Keeler et al., 1988). Since not all the care military beneficiaries receive is from MTFs and therefore free, the effects of cost sharing on military utilization would be less than those for families in the experiment.

There are other possible explanations for the higher health care utilization rates found in the military population; one centers on different patterns of medical practice in the military. The health literature contains many studies that document the variability of medical practice, for example, by geographic area. In the military, there is some incentive to increase utilization because MTF resources are determined by historical utilization levels. A comparison of military and civilian practice patterns is, however, well beyond the scope of this study; thus, we mention practice patterns only as a possibility. Other potential explanations derive from the military's emphasis on good health, which may encourage broader health care use, as well as from family separations, which may lead active-duty spouses to more frequently seek medical advice, especially for their children.

Military Utilization by Health Care Source: MHSS Data Versus the Beneficiary Survey

Military beneficiaries have three major sources of care: MTFs, CHAMPUS, and non-MHSS sources. The beneficiary survey asked for visits and days of hospitalization according to the location of care: (1) an MTF or PRIMUS/NAVCARE clinic; (2) a civilian hospital, doctor's office, or clinic; or (3) a Veterans Administration (VA) hospital or clinic or other source. The survey also asked whether CHAMPUS paid for any portion of the civilian care used, although it did not ask how many of the reported visits and days were covered—information that is available from CHAMPUS claims data.[5] The survey is, however, the only source of data on total civilian utilization. To examine military utilization by source of care, we therefore looked both at the survey data and at regularly collected MHSS data. These two data sets yielded differences that have implications for other analyses of military utilization. The remainder of this section describes the MHSS data sources we used, the mix of health care sources used according to the survey and MHSS data, and the differences we found between the two types of data.

MHSS Data Systems

The MHSS maintains a number of data systems that can be used to estimate health care utilization rates. Since these data omit civilian care not financed by CHAMPUS and care obtained through other government programs (e.g., Medicare and the VA), however, they offer an incomplete record of utilization for many military beneficiaries. The beneficiary survey data are more comprehensive and, as discussed earlier, more comparable to the data provided by civilian surveys. Such survey data are, however, subject to a number of biases. Our original intent in comparing these two data sources was to assess incompleteness in the MHSS data and bias in the survey data—but in carrying out this comparison, we uncovered a number of other problems in the MHSS data that, if not corrected, render such data inadequate to the task of measuring utilization rates even for MHSS services.

Calculating Utilization Rates Using MHSS Data Systems

Per-capita utilization rates can be estimated by dividing aggregate utilization by the number of beneficiaries generating that utilization. Accurate estimates

---

[5]Respondents cannot usually provide this kind of information in a self-administered survey.

require accurate utilization and beneficiary population data; in particular, the utilization measure must be for the same beneficiaries included in the population data. A method that is more difficult but that ensures a match between utilization and population involves the averaging of data collected for individual beneficiaries. Since MTF outpatient data are not reported for individuals, however, only the first method can be used with routinely collected MHSS data.

The Defense Medical Information System (DMIS) is the principal source of routinely collected data on the MHSS. Within DMIS, the following sources provide the data needed to calculate utilization rates:

- The Defense Eligibility Enrollment Reporting System (DEERS) records basic information on each eligible beneficiary and reports beneficiary counts by geographic area. The FY92 counts we used to calculate utilization rates correct the DEERS counts for (1) new ZIP codes in several catchment areas; (2) fluctuations in the active-duty population at training facilities such that counts reflect average training loads; and (3) mislocation of some active-duty dependents.[6]

- Two data systems—biometrics and the Medical Expense and Performance Reporting System (MEPRS)—record MTF utilization. As part of the biometrics data system, the MTFs generate a summary discharge record for each hospitalized patient; thus, patient-level data are available for inpatient utilization. However, that is not the case for outpatient utilization. The biometrics and MEPRS data systems also include annual counts by MTF of outpatient visits, admissions and/or discharges, and inpatient days. These counts are reported by clinical service or beneficiary category, although the data for CHAMPUS- and Medicare-eligible retired beneficiaries are combined and survivors and other beneficiaries are combined with retired dependents.

- CHAMPUS utilization is recorded on extracts of the individual claims submitted for payment. Quarterly summary reports display data assembled three months after the end of the fiscal year; since not all the claims have been submitted by that date, the CHAMPUS office estimates that the reports are only about 88 percent complete.

_____

[6]In 1992, DEERS showed almost double the number of overseas active-duty dependents as in previous years and an offsetting decline in active-duty dependents in the United States (especially in noncatchment areas). The change reflected new rules for locating dependents lacking a recent address. Our analysis of the survey data and other data sources suggested that the new rules incorrectly located enough dependents of active-duty personnel on unaccompanied assignments to noticeably bias non-catchment-area and some catchment-area population counts.

Outpatient Utilization by Source of Care

Since MTF services are less available in noncatchment areas and since the use of some civilian services may be lower in catchment areas, we sought to identify the sources of care used in both types of areas. From the survey, we can easily tie outpatient visits by source of care (e.g., MTF, civilian, or other) to individuals, thus allowing us to estimate average visits by source for both catchment-area and non-catchment-area populations. The MHSS data can support a similar calculation for CHAMPUS visits but not for MTF visits; we must therefore assume that outpatient visits at military hospitals are made by local catchment-area beneficiaries and that visits at outlying clinics are made by non-catchment-area beneficiaries. The result is a misestimation of the true utilization rates in both areas. Estimates of non-CHAMPUS civilian visits and other government visits are available only from the survey.

Figures 4 to 7 show the average number of visits recorded for the major beneficiary groups in the MHSS data in FY92 and in the survey in early FY93. Here we provide information for beneficiaries age 65 and over in addition to the other groups. The figures lead us to two general conclusions about the use of outpatient services, as measured by the two data sources. First, the military beneficiary groups rely to a varying extent on MTFs to meet their health care demands. Second, routinely collected MHSS data generate higher estimates of use than the survey shows. The difference is especially large for active-duty personnel and for MTF outpatient use.

Active-duty personnel obtain essentially all their health care from MTFs, whether or not they live in a catchment area; for the vast majority of active-duty dependents who live in a catchment area (87 percent), MTFs provide at least three-fourths of their outpatient care. Those living in other areas report that they do use MTFs; making one-third of their visits to such facilities. Retirees and their dependents of all ages are least reliant on MTFs for outpatient care, those living in catchment areas obtain half or more of their care from MTFs, but in noncatchment areas the civilian sector provides most outpatient care. Finally, military beneficiaries' utilization of VA and other providers' outpatient services is limited. Military retirees report that they make only about 5 percent of their visits to VA clinics.

Differences in MTF Visit Rates by Data Source. MTF visit rates estimated from MHSS data for catchment-area beneficiaries are considerably higher than survey estimates (the bottom portions of the bars in Figures 4 to 7). Non-catchment-area clinics also record high visit rates for their active-duty population, but the visit rates for other beneficiaries are low in relation to survey estimates. As

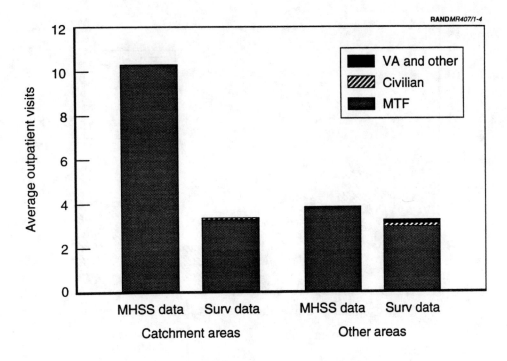

Figure 4—Active-Duty Outpatient Use by Source

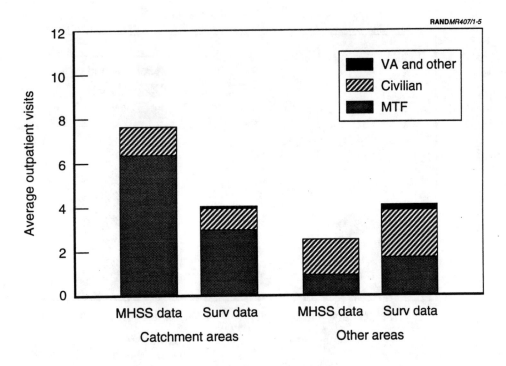

Figure 5—Active-Duty Dependent Outpatient Use by Source

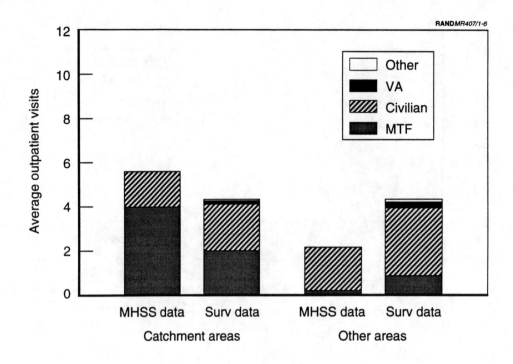

Figure 6—Retiree/Dependent/Survivor Under 65 Outpatient Use by Source

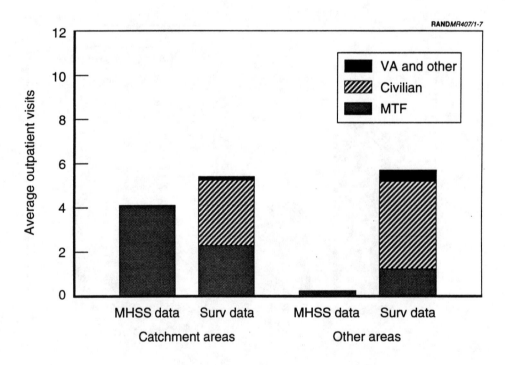

Figure 7—Medicare Outpatient Use by Source

mentioned earlier, we were unable to verify that the population DEERS records for a catchment area is the population that is making the visits recorded by the MHSS data. Therefore, we believe that the catchment-area and non-catchment-area rates are misestimated; most probably, the former are overestimated and the latter underestimated. If we combine the areas to eliminate these locational problems, the MTF visit rates estimated from MHSS data are higher than the survey estimates by 200 percent for active-duty personnel, 90 percent for active-duty dependents, 70 percent for retirees, survivors, and dependents under age 65, and 50 percent for over-65 beneficiaries.

The differences in MTF visit rates measured from MHSS data and survey data probably result from errors in both data sources. The survey data underestimate the number of outpatient visits for two reasons. First, numerous studies have shown that recall bias causes mail-survey respondents to underestimate outpatient use by approximately 20 percent (Jobe et al., 1990; Siemiatycki, 1979; Yaffe et al., 1978). Second, adding to the effects of recall bias is this survey's design, which limits the number of visits that can be reported for each person to 10. In their report on the survey, Lurie et al. (1994) estimated what the visit rates would be without this limitation. A comparison of our survey estimates, which are unadjusted, with the survey report's adjusted estimates indicates that our estimates are as much as 15 percent too low. Since these two error sources taken together account for less than a 40 percent difference, however, other factors must play a role as well.

The differences in MTF utilization rates measured from MHSS data and the survey also reflect varying criteria for defining a visit and probably an incentive to overreport MTF utilization. MHSS data systems treat each outpatient encounter as a visit; the survey asked about visits "to a doctor or an assistant." Some examples of encounters that are recorded as visits in the MHSS data but not necessarily in the survey responses include picking up a prescription refill from a clinic, a telephone inquiry, immediate follow-up care, or a telephone consultation with a second provider or clinic. Moreover, because funding of almost all MTFs during FY92 was based on historical workload, such facilities had an incentive to be as inclusive as possible in counting outpatient visits.

Other possible reasons for the differences include (1) incorrect recall of the location of a visit (MTF versus civilian) by some in the survey; and (2) use of a survey sample that is not fully representative of the beneficiary population from which it was drawn. Included in the first category would be misidentification of PRIMUS and NAVCARE clinic visits, which we include in the MTF counts as civilian visits.

Differences in Civilian/Other Visit Rates by Data Source. The only source of data we had on civilian utilization for active-duty personnel and Medicare-eligible beneficiaries was the survey. For the other beneficiaries, MHSS data systems record civilian utilization only if it is financed at least in part by CHAMPUS; by contrast, the survey asked for all civilian utilization, regardless of the payer. Few active-duty dependents have other insurance, but just over half of all retirees and dependents under age 65 report having other coverage. Thus, the civilian visit rates calculated from MHSS data are similar to the survey-based rates for active-duty dependents but are lower for other beneficiaries.

A comparison of the MHSS data on civilian care, which includes services obtained only through CHAMPUS, with the survey will yield an imprecise estimate of the CHAMPUS share of civilian care. The ratio of CHAMPUS visits to total civilian visits reported in the survey is actually above 1.00 for active-duty dependents and .70 for retirees and their dependents—.80 in catchment areas but only .60 in noncatchment areas.

Inpatient Utilization Rates by Source of Care

From the survey, we calculated the fraction of beneficiaries hospitalized for at least one night during a 12-month period. CHAMPUS routinely reports the number of beneficiaries with hospital claims. We counted the number of beneficiaries hospitalized in MTFs from individual patient records, separating catchment-area residents from non-catchment-area residents using the ZIP codes listed in the records. Figures 8 to 11 plot these admission probabilities.[7] Estimates of civilian hospitalizations not financed by CHAMPUS and other government hospitalizations are available only from the survey.

The mix of sources of care used by each beneficiary group for inpatient care generally resembles that used for outpatient care. However, active-duty personnel report getting more inpatient than outpatient care from civilian providers, especially in noncatchment areas. As far as we can tell, these civilian hospitalizations are not recorded in MHSS data systems. The other notable difference in the mix of inpatient and outpatient sources lies in the heavier use of VA and other services for inpatient care; almost 10 percent of Medicare-eligible recipients reporting some hospital use in the survey list the source as "other."

---

[7]We did not estimate utilization rates for National Guard and Reserve personnel. A match of the MTF inpatient and DEERS records showed that only about one-fourth of those hospitalized are listed in DEERS. Therefore, the utilization and population counts are not comparable. If we had the patient-level visit data to perform a similar check, we would expect to find the same mismatch.

23

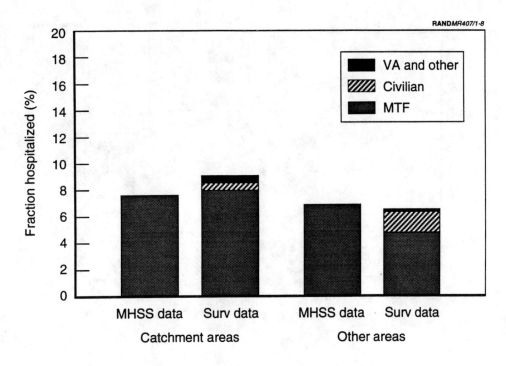

Figure 8—Active-Duty Inpatient Use by Source

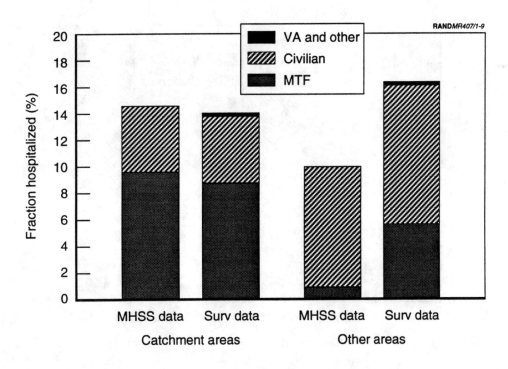

Figure 9—Active-Duty Dependent Inpatient Use by Source

24

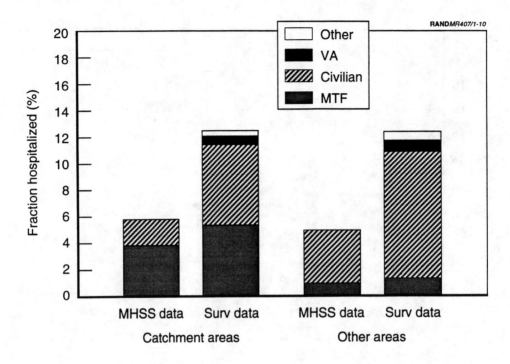

Figure 10—Retiree/Dependent/Survivor Under 65 Inpatient Use by Source

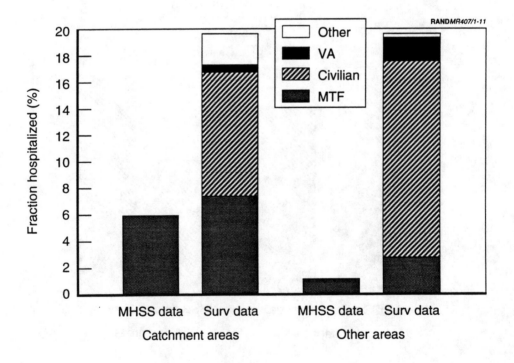

Figure 11—Medicare Inpatient Use by Source

Differences in MTF Hospitalization Rates by Data Source. The two estimates of MTF use are more similar for catchment-area populations of active-duty personnel and their dependents than for non-catchment-area populations. Further investigation showed that replacing the ZIP codes listed in the MTF inpatient data with the ZIP codes in DEERS decreases the number of hospitalizations attributed to non-catchment-area residents by two-thirds for active-duty personnel while increasing it by one-third for active-duty dependents. While this is sufficient to lower the active-duty hospitalization rate to a level below the survey estimate, it eliminates only some of the difference in the estimates for active-duty dependents. The ZIP-code source used to assign location makes less difference for retirees and other beneficiaries and for all beneficiaries in catchment areas.

If problems in locating beneficiaries are the principal source of the sizable differences in inpatient estimates in noncatchment areas, such differences should disappear if we combine the two types of areas. The fractions hospitalized in all areas measured with the two data sources are within 3 percent for active-duty personnel and 10 percent for their dependents, but the MHSS-based rates are only 70 percent of the survey-based rates for retirees and their dependents. Possible explanations for the difference for this last group include (1) recall bias in the survey, with respondents reporting some hospitalizations that occurred more than one year previously; (2) incorrect recall of the location of hospitalization (MTF versus civilian) by some in the survey; (3) survey respondents counting nonovernight hospitalizations; and (4) a nonrepresentative survey sample.

Differences in Civilian/Other Hospitalization Rates. The estimates of civilian hospital use derived from CHAMPUS records and from the survey are similar for active-duty dependents, although the fraction of non-catchment-area residents with an MTF hospitalization may be underestimated in the MHSS data. For other CHAMPUS eligibles, the ratio of the fraction with CHAMPUS hospital use to that reporting any civilian use in the survey is under 40 percent overall— 33 percent in catchment areas and 40 percent in noncatchment areas.[8] Even if we consider the "extra" MTF hospitalizations reported for catchment-area residents in the survey to be mistaken civilian hospitalizations, the fraction of those residents with a CHAMPUS hospitalization is at most 50 percent of the survey-based civilian hospitalization rate for retirees, survivors, and their dependents under age 65. Thus, the CHAMPUS share of these beneficiaries' civilian care is

---

[8]CHAMPUS cannot be used by Medicare-age beneficiaries, so we do not report CHAMPUS use in Figure 11.

considerably smaller for inpatient than for outpatient services, probably because CHAMPUS inpatient benefits are less generous in relation to civilian plans. Beneficiaries with other insurance will often find it covers most inpatient costs but that they must turn to CHAMPUS to fill in gaps in outpatient coverage—especially for mental health and preventive care.

4. Analytic Cases Developed to Study Demand in the MHSS

Numerous potential alternatives exist for restructuring the MHSS. Only a small number of alternatives were chosen as analytic cases for this study. The four principal analytic cases examined are:

1. A managed-care program like the one currently being implemented (the baseline case);

2. Maximum practicable health care provision in MTFs;

3. Minimum health care provision in MTFs with two options:

   a. Provision of only reception and referral centers in U.S. military hospitals during wartime, augmented by care in civilian and Veterans Administration hospitals, or

   b. Provision of all required care in U.S. military hospitals; and

4. Military-civilian competition in providing health care, with a choice of MTF HMOs and civilian HMO and fee-for-service (FFS)/PPO options.

Table 4 summarizes the health plans that would be available to beneficiaries in each case. In addition to varying the number and size of military health care facilities, the cases vary how the MHSS structures health plans using MTFs and civilian providers. The current system, with its managed-care reforms, employs a structure that is retained in the second ("maximum military") case—one that combines in one or more health plans both MTFs and civilian providers, with care from the latter financed through a health-insurance program like CHAMPUS. The reform programs introduce a second health plan that beneficiaries may choose instead of the traditional option. This managed-care option combines MTFs with a much smaller civilian provider network, manages patients more aggressively, and offers beneficiaries enhanced benefits in return for more restricted provider choice. The third ("minimum military") case replaces this structure with civilian health plans for non-active-duty beneficiaries. The fourth case would allow beneficiaries to choose between an MTF-based plan and one or more commercial civilian plans. In this case, the MTFs are converted to military HMOs that are responsible for providing all care to enrolled beneficiaries either through their own staffs or through civilian

Table 4

Health Plan Options Across the Analytic Cases

Case	Health Plan Options
1. Managed-care (baseline case)	In hospital catchment areas and most clinic service areas: the current MTF/CHAMPUS system with a managed-care enrollment option in all catchment areas
	In other areas: CHAMPUS
2. Maximum MTF	Same as case 1, but with more military hospitals, expanded beds at military hospitals that are particularly short, and expanded staffing at most hospitals
3. Minimum MTF	For active duty: direct provision of care at or through MTFs, many of which would be primary care clinics
	For other beneficiaries: commercial health plan(s)
4. Military-civilian competition	In hospital catchment areas and some clinic service areas: beneficiaries choose an MTF-based HMO or commercial plan. MTFs arrange all medical services for their enrollees and provide no services for commercial plan enrollees
	Outside these areas: beneficiaries choose a commercial plan.

contractors. Beneficiaries have the choice of enrolling in this military HMO or in a commercial health care plan. This case therefore places MTFs in direct competition for beneficiary enrollment with the civilian market, which is not true of the first three cases. Although it was developed before the President's health reform plans, this case generally describes the choices military beneficiaries are expected to have when national health reform is implemented.

Base closures and personnel drawdowns will continue to affect the MHSS until 1997 and possibly beyond. In light of these ongoing changes, we have specified two versions of the cases. The first is based on the current MTF system and beneficiary population, and the second incorporates the changes expected in both of these variables by 1997.[1]

The remainder of this section describes each of the cases in sufficient detail to support a broad analysis. Obviously, many details that would be necessary to actually implement the changes outlined in these cases are omitted by the scope of this report.

---

[1]We based the 1997 estimates on planned base closures and the recent DoD "bottom-up review."

The Current Managed-Care Case (#1)

As was described in Sec. 2, DoD is gradually implementing a managed-care program that is based on the CRI model.[2] This program would offer beneficiaries the choice of (1) the standard MTF/CHAMPUS plan along with an optional PPO that would offer discounts for beneficiaries who chose selected civilian providers or (2) an HMO that would combine military and selected civilian providers.[3] In addition to offering lower-cost shares, the HMO plan would cover some additional services (e.g., adult preventive care). The proposed benefit package for the two plans is shown in Table 5.

Other key components of the current managed-care case include:

- Assignment of beneficiaries who choose the HMO to a primary care provider who serves as a "gatekeeper" to specialty care.

Table 5

Overview of Current Managed-Care Benefits for Civilian Care

	Active-Duty Dependents		Retirees and Dependents
	Jr. Enlisted	Other	
Standard plan			
Annual premium	$0	$0	$0
Deductible	$50/person; $150/family	$100/person; $300/family	$100/person; $300/family
Outpatient copayment	20%	20%	25%
Inpatient copayment	$9.30/day or $25[a]	$9.30/day or $25[a]	25% or $265/day[b]
Enrollment option			
Annual premium	0	$35/person; $70/family	$50/person; $100/family
Deductible	0	0	0
Outpatient clinic fee	$5/visit	$10/visit	$15/visit
Inpatient copayment	$9.30/day or $25[a]	$9.30/day or $25[a]	25% or $125/day[b]

[a]Whichever is larger.
[b]Whichever is less.

---

[2]In reality, this alternative would also incorporate capitation budgeting, which is currently being implemented. Until recently, most MTF resources have been allocated based on the MTFs' workloads during the previous year. OSD has directed that in FY94 all MTFs receive a budget based on the number of MHSS users they serve. If strictly enforced, capitation budgeting should alter future utilization patterns and costs in this alternative. However, we have not incorporated capitation budgets because at this early stage we would be guessing at the changes that would occur. In the final version of the report, we will indicate how we expect capitation budgeting might affect our results.

[3]Actually, beneficiaries would automatically be enrolled in the first option unless they voluntarily enrolled in the HMO.

- A health care "finder service" that refers enrolled patients in need of specialized care to the most cost-effective providers and that may provide general referral information to nonenrolled patients.

- Quality assurance (QA) and utilization review (UR) programs to ensure that the care provided is appropriate, of high quality, and delivered in the most cost-effective setting.

The managed-care plan would be provided at 117 hospitals at the end of 1992 and at the 101 military hospitals that will remain open after BRAC 3 in 1997. Table 6 lists these hospitals. The managed-care plan might also be offered in areas served by a number of outlying military clinics. However, a managed-care plan may be impractical in some of these clinic areas, and there are insufficient data for predicting the costs for managed-care programs in clinic areas. In areas without an MTF, we have assumed that this case would offer only the standard plan.

The Maximum-MTF Case (#2)

The maximum-MTF case has the same basic structure and benefit package as that defined for the managed-care case, but features an expanded number of military hospitals and an increase in the size and staffing of existing military hospitals. To lend practicality to this case, we established a minimum-size criterion for adding new hospitals: that the catchment-area beneficiary population must support at least 70 beds.[4] In determining where to add facilities, we considered:

- The size of the non-Medicare beneficiary population. We determined that roughly 1.5 beds per 1,000 beneficiaries represented a reasonable planning factor for determining hospital size.[5]

---

[4]Inasmuch as the research literature on hospital economies of scale inadequately adjusts for patient mix and other cost factors, it is difficult to determine whether small hospitals are in fact inefficient. However, we decided not to consider very small hospitals because the literature does suggest that quality improves with volume in hospitals, and it seemed unlikely that constructing small hospitals serving few beneficiaries would appreciably decrease MHSS costs. See Luft et al. (1979), Luft (1980), and Keeler et al. (1992).

[5]HMOs typically use fewer than 2 beds per 1,000 enrollees. The estimate of 2 beds per 1,000 is compatible with the assumptions that the population under 65 years of age uses 350 hospital days per year per 1,000 enrollees and that the population 65 or older uses 2,430 days per 1,000; see Kronick et al. (1993). By way of comparison, in 1990 the military operated about 1.7 beds per 1,000 non-Medicare beneficiaries. To calculate this figure, we used workload by beneficiary category to allocate 85 percent of the MTFs' 14,000 beds to this population. Hospitals with 70 or more beds that are not medical centers operated 1.5 beds per 1,000 (with an interquartile range of 1.3 to 1.8). Given our principal interest of adding facilities of this type, we used 1.5 beds per 1,000 non-Medicare beneficiaries as our planning factor.

Table 6

Military Hospitals for the Managed-Care Case

Hospital	Year 92	Year 97	Hospital	Year 92	Year 97	Hospital	Year 92	Year 97
Redstone Arsl, AL	H	H	Patrick AFB, FL	H	H	Ft. Bragg, NC	H	H
Ft. McClellan, AL	H	H	Ft. Gordon, GA	H	H	Seymour Jnsn, NC	H	H
Ft. Rucker, AL	H	H	Ft. Benning, GA	H	H	Camp Lejeune, NC	H	H
Maxwell AFB, AL	H	H	Ft. Stewart, GA	H	H	Cherry Point, NC	H	H
Ft. Wainwright, AK	H	H	Moody AFB, GA	H	H	Grand Forks, ND	H	H
Elmendorf AFB, AK	H	H	Robins AFB, GA	H	H	Minot AFB, ND	H	H
Adak NH, AK	H	H	Ft. Shafter, HI	H	H	Wright-Patt, OH	H	H
Ft. Huachuca, AZ	H	H	Mountain Hme, ID	H	H	Tinker AFB, OK	H	H
Luke AFB, AZ	H	H	Chanute AFB, IL	H		Altus AFB, OK	H	H
Davis Monthan, AZ	H	H	Scott AFB, IL	H	H	Ft. Sill, OK	H	H
Little Rock, AR	H	H	Great Lakes, IL	H	H	Newport NH, RI	H	H
Travis AFB, CA	H	H	Ft. Ben Hrrsn, IN	H		Shaw AFB, SC	H	H
Beale AFB, CA	H	H	Ft. Riley, KS	H	H	Charlestn NH, SC	H	H
McClellan AFB, CA	H	H	Ft. Leavnwrth, KS	H	H	Beaufort NH, SC	H	H
Castle AFB, CA	H		Ft. Campbell, KY	H	H	Ft. Jackson, SC	H	H
Vandenbrg AFB, CA	H	H	Ft. Knox, KY	H	H	Ellswrth AFB, SD	H	H
Edwards AFB, CA	H	H	Barksdle AFB, LA	H	H	Millingtn NH, TN	H	H
March AFB, CA	H	C	Ft. Polk, LA	H	H	Ft. Bliss, TX	H	H
Presidio, CA	H	C	Loring AFB, ME	H		Ft. Sam Hstn, TX	H	H
Ft. Ord, CA	H	C	Andrews AFB, MD	H	H	Ft. Hood, TX	H	H
Camp Pendletn, CA	H	H	Bethesda NH, MD	H	H	Reese AFB, TX	H	H
Long Beach NH, CA	H	C	Patuxent Rvr, MD	H	H	Dyess AFB, TX	H	H
Oakland NH, CA	H	C	Ft. Meade, MD	H	H	Sheppard AFB, TX	H	H
Lemoore NH, CA	H	H	Ft. Devens, MA	H	C	Laughlin AFB, TX	H	H
San Diego NH, CA	H	H	K.I. Sawyer, MI	H		Bergstrm AFB, TX	H	
29 Palms, CA	H	H	Keesler AFB, MS	H	H	Carswell AFB, TX	H	
Ft. Irwin, CA	H	H	Columbus AFB, MS	H	H	Lackland AFB, TX	H	H
Fitzsmmns AMC, CO	H	H	Ft. Leonrd Wd, MO	H	H	Corpus Chsti, TX	H	H
Ft. Carson, CO	H	H	Whiteman AFB, MO	H	H	Hill AFB, UT	H	H
USAF Academy, CO	H	H	Offutt AFB, NE	H	H	Langley AFB, VA	H	H
Groton NH, CT	H	H	Nellis AFB, NV	H	H	Ft. Eustis, VA	H	H
Dover AFB, DE	H	H	Ft. Monmouth, NJ	H	H	Ft. Lee, VA	H	H
WR-Washington, DC	H	H	McGuire AFB, NJ	H	H	Ft. Belvoir, VA	H	H
Pensacola NH, FL	H	H	Kirtland AFB, NM	H	H	Portsmouth, VA	H	H
Jacksonville, FL	H	H	Holloman AFB, NM	H	H	Ft. Lewis, WA	H	H
Orlando NH, FL	H	C	Cannon AFB, NM	H	H	Bremerton NH, WA	H	H
Eglin AFB, FL	H	H	West Point, NY	H	H	Oak Harbor, WA	H	H
Tyndall AFB,FL	H	H	Plattsburg, NY	H		Fairchld AFB, WA	H	H
MacDill AFB, FL	H	H	Griffiss AFB, NY	H	C	FE Warrn AFB, WY	H	H

NOTE: An "H" means hospital, while a "C" means clinic only.

- Providing the military hospitals enough capacity to allow Medicare beneficiaries the same MTF access that they currently enjoy. This access varies significantly with the service and with the size of the military hospitals; we added 1.9 beds per 1,000 Medicare beneficiaries, the average for DoD's midsize hospitals.[6]

- Increasing the physician-to-bed ratio for most hospitals up to the 90th-percentile level.

These factors imply that we would establish new hospitals in areas where at least 47,000 noncatchment, non-Medicare military beneficiaries are located within a 40-mile catchment area, with a smaller threshold in cases where Medicare beneficiaries require a significant number of beds. We found seven areas in which the beneficiary numbers in the late 1990s will meet this criterion, as shown in Table 7. With the exception of Atlanta, the one area that qualified for the addition of a military hospital in 1992, all of these areas are served by military hospitals that will be closed between 1992 and 1997. The areas that fall just below our criterion in 1997 are New York, New York (54 beds), Miami, Florida (49 beds), Harrisburg, Pennsylvania (44 beds), New Orleans, Louisiana (43 beds), Austin, Texas (43 beds), and Monterey, California (40 beds).

Table 7

Added Military Hospitals in Maximum-MTF Case

City	St.	Hospital	Total	Medicare	Non-Medicare Active Duty	Non-Medicare Active-Duty Dependents	Non-Medicare Retirees/ Dependents
1997							
Los Angeles	CA	West L.A. VA	122	38	15	22	47
San Bernardino	CA	March AFB	85	30	4	6	45
San Francisco	CA	Presidio	74	30	6	7	31
Orlando	FL	Orlando NTC	82	33	2	2	45
Atlanta	GA	Ft. McPherson	83	20	6	14	43
Boston	MA	S. Boston VA	86	23	12	18	33
Dallas	TX	Carswell AFB	99	26	3	6	64
1992							
Atlanta	GA	Ft. McPherson	99	19	9	22	49

_____

[6]In FY90, medium-size MTFs averaged 1.3 occupied beds per 1,000 Medicare beneficiaries, with the interquartile range running from 0.8 to 3.1 (Navy MTFs averaged considerably fewer beds occupied by Medicare beneficiaries than Army and Air Force MTFs). On average, the medium-size MTFs averaged 0.69 bed occupied per operating bed. Dividing the 1.3 by the 0.69 yields the required number of beds per 1,000 Medicare beneficiaries.

In some cases, MTFs might also be expanded to better serve the beneficiary populations. We expanded MTFs if they met the following criteria: (1) if the beneficiary population could support at least 70 beds; (2) if a substantial expansion of the MTF is indicated, i.e., the capacity needed for the non-Medicare population must be at least half again the current capacity; and (3) if the catchment area did not noticeably overlap with that of another MTF.[7] We used the criterion of 1.5 beds per 1,000 non-Medicare beneficiaries to determine which hospitals to add or expand, but we also included 1.9 beds per 1,000 Medicare beneficiaries in establishing the number of beds for each of these hospitals. Table 8 shows these bed criteria.[8] The resulting list of hospitals warranting expansion totals 16 in 1992 and 13 in 1997, as shown in Table 9 (where the category of "beds required" includes both non-Medicare and Medicare beds).

We also examined the current staffing at the military hospitals and determined that there were substantial variations in full-time equivalents (FTEs) per operating bed. Many hospitals might well be better able to serve military beneficiaries if their physician levels were simply increased. We decided to increase the FTEs per bed up to the 90th-percentile level, which in FY92 was 1.2 FTEs per bed in small hospitals and 0.9 FTE per bed in medium-size hospitals and medical centers.

In developing this case, we also considered increasing the number of military clinics located in noncatchment areas. In FY92, there were 74 of these clinics. Using a criterion of at least 5,000 military beneficiaries within a 20-mile service

Table 8

FY90 Bed Requirements per 1,000 Medicare Beneficiaries

Service	Medium-Size MTFs			Medical Centers		
	Beds Occupied	Avg. Census	Beds Reqd.	Beds Occupied	Avg. Census	Beds Reqd.
Army	2.5	82%	3.0	8.2	81%	10.0
Air Force	1.6	67%	2.4	8.0	69%	11.6
Navy	0.6	55%	1.15	2.8	62%	4.5

---

[7]Both Fort Belvoir and Fort Meade would otherwise be on the expansion list, but many of the beneficiaries from their catchment areas actually receive care at either Walter Reed Army Medical Center or Bethesda Naval Hospital, and this pattern would likely continue even if Fort Belvoir's and Fort Meade's operating capacities were expanded.

[8]We used the average bed usage per 1,000 Medicare beneficiaries rather than current usage at the specific facilities because as these facilities expand, we would expect them to provide a wider range of medical specialists and thus to require that fewer Medicare beneficiaries be referred to other MTFs (especially medical centers).

Table 9

Military Hospitals with Likely Expansion Requirements

| Hospital | St. | Current Operating Beds | Beds Required | | | Expanded Wartime Beds |
			Medical Center	Other	Total	
1997						
Luke AFB	AZ	55	29	77	106	190
Travis AFB	CA	220	241	111	352	480
McClellan AFB	CA	35	28	73	101	106
Camp Pendleton	CA	128	50	195	245	624
San Diego NH	CA	393	273	381	654	764
MacDill AFB	FL	55	53	92	145	150
Patrick AFB	FL	15	23	49	72	83
Scott AFB	IL	115	78	68	146	422
Offutt AFB	NE	50	6	70	76	123
Nellis AFB	NV	35	12	66	78	50
McGuire AFB	NJ	36	31	100	131	617
Tinker AFB	OK	25	13	62	75	90
Ft. Hood	TX	126	8	174	182	1770
1992						
Luke AFB	AZ	55	32	63	95	190
Davis Mon AFB	AZ	35	19	53	72	112
McClellan AFB	CA	35	31	83	115	106
March AFB	CA	80	31	81	111	190
Long Beach	CA	120	30	166	196	692[a]
MacDill AFB	FL	55	59	111	170	150
Patrick AFB	FL	15	25	52	77	83
Scott AFB	IL	115	69	89	158	422
Ft. Devens	MA	35	35	70	106	116[a]
Offutt AFB	NE	50	7	74	81	123
Nellis AFB	NV	35	16	76	91	50
McGuire AFB	NJ	36	43	101	145	617
Ft. Bragg	NC	206	61	222	283	400
Tinker AFB	OK	25	15	74	89	90
Ft. Eustis	VA	42	11	66	78	100
Ft. Lee	VA	52	16	56	73	121

[a]Numbers from 1988.

area, we identified 41 additional locations for military clinics. However, for reasons discussed in the next section, we did not include the added clinics in the final version of this case.

The Minimum-MTF Case (#3)

The minimum-MTF case attempts to shift as many military beneficiaries as possible to civilian health care while retaining the military's capacity to perform its wartime medical mission. The facilities and staff required for the wartime mission are employed in peacetime to provide primary care for active-duty personnel. Since active-duty workloads may be inadequate to fill the facilities and maintain the skills of military personnel, this case incorporates strategies for employing any excess capacity.

Civilian Health Plans

In this case, DoD would select from among the large number of civilian health plans available within the United States. Although some plans combine features from more than one type, these are of three major types:

- Fee-for-service plans, which historically have dominated the civilian market. These plans cover services obtained from any health care provider, with payment made according to the nature and extent of the services provided. Today, most FFS plans incorporate some managed-care features, such as prior authorization for hospital treatment.

- Preferred-provider organization plans, which modify FFS plans by establishing a network of providers who negotiate discounted payment rates and agree to submit their treatment decisions to utilization review. Most PPOs are "point of service"—that is to say, plan members may elect to use a network or a nonnetwork provider at the point of service. If members do elect to use the network, the plan usually pays a higher fraction of the cost and may cover some services that would not otherwise be covered.

- Health maintenance organization plans that were developed many years ago. The key feature of an HMO resides in its payment mechanism; unlike FFS and PPO plans, payment is per capita (per patient) rather than per service, and the patient's choice of provider is limited. There are two major types of HMOs. The first, independent practice associations (IPAs), contract with physicians in private practice; primary care physicians (e.g., family practitioners and pediatricians) receive a per-capita payment, and specialists and hospitals are paid per service. The second, group-model and staff-model HMOs, effectively employ their own providers and usually maintain hospitals. These two types of HMOs differ only in the way their providers are organized.

As Figure 12 shows, PPOs enjoy a large share of the civilian market. FFS plans are available everywhere, but PPOs and HMOs are not found in rural areas or even in some small cities. DoD could, however, encourage PPOs and HMOs to

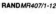

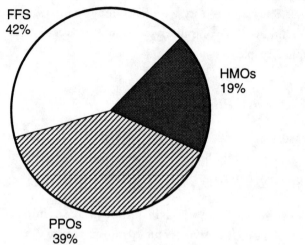

Figure 12—Shares of the Current Civilian Health Care Market

operate in areas with sizable military populations, and these plans are likely in any event to spread with national health reform.

Benefit Package

Under the minimum-MTF case, active-duty personnel would continue to receive free comprehensive care at or through military facilities. The benefits for other beneficiaries would depend on the type of civilian plan chosen. This case was specified to be consistent with the current MHSS benefit package. FFS plans are assumed to require the same cost sharing and to cover the same services that CHAMPUS does now. As in CRI and the FI-PPO program, use of an optional PPO in these plans would lower the coinsurance rate by five percentage points. HMO plans would have the same benefits as the managed-care enrollment option in cases 1 and 2; this would mean that standard HMO packages would have to be modified, particularly to expand mental health benefits.[9]

MTFs Needed to Meet Wartime Requirements

We define two options for meeting the wartime military bed requirement in the United States. In the first option (reception and referral), military facilities would serve as reception facilities for casualties being returned to the United States,

---

[9]National health reform would lead to changes in the benefit packages in civilian plans and probably in the MHSS as well.

provide some casualties with additional treatment, and refer the remainder to civilian or Veterans Administration hospitals. This option would maintain six military hospitals to fulfill this requirement, all located near military airlift bases and balanced both geographically and along service lines, as shown in Table 10.[10] We also assume that Dover will remain a major airlift base on the East Coast, but since its hospital is so small, we have added Walter Reed as the major medical center close to Dover to provide in-depth reception ability. In neither list are the hospitals definitive; if others were chosen instead, however, there would be little change in the analysis.

The second option (military care) provides a sufficient number of military hospitals to meet the wartime bed requirements for CONUS care within the expanded bed capacities of the hospitals;[11] these hospitals are also distributed across the United States to allow recovering casualties to be as close to family members as possible. The list of hospitals in Table 10 generally includes newer and better-equipped facilities.[12] The 1992 and 1997 versions of this case include the same list of hospitals.

Under this concept, the 11 hospitals identified in Table 10 would provide most of the care for active-duty personnel in their catchment areas and would likely expand the services they provide to military personnel from other areas. In addition, as discussed below, they could provide care for non-active-duty beneficiaries under contract to the civilian health plans that cover these beneficiaries. At other military bases that now have military hospitals (listed in Table 11), only a clinic facility would be retained to care for active-duty personnel.

In setting up this case, we required that an outlying clinic have a noncatchment population of 1,600 active-duty personnel to remain open.[13] This would mean closing 57 of the 74 outlying clinics existing in FY92.

---

[10]Bethesda Naval Hospital is not included in either of the options. Although the capabilities of this facility cannot be disputed, there does not appear to be a wartime need for two medical centers in the Washington, D.C., area.

[11]The overall DoD requirement is somewhat less than the service-specific bed requirements because the timing of the service requirements differs among services. The Army and Navy totals from this list are somewhat less than their service-specific requirements given the lower DoD total.

[12]An even more radical option would be to ignore the service-specific bed requirements and simply choose the best military hospitals regardless of their service. Such an approach would yield only a few changes from the list in Table 10.

[13]In some cases, we list a clinic even though DEERS does not show the required number of personnel because current active-duty workloads suggest that the population estimates are in error.

Table 10

Military Hospitals, Minimum-MTF Case

Reception-and-Referral		Military Care	
Hospital	St.	Hospital	St.
San Diego NH	CA	San Diego NH	CA
Dover AFB	DE	WRAMC-Washington	DC
WRAMC-Washington	DC	Jacksonville NH	FL
Lackland AFB	TX	Ft. Shafter	HI
Portsmouth NH	VA	Ft. Campbell	KY
Ft. Lewis	WA	Ft. Bragg	NC
		Camp Lejeune	NC
		Ft. Hood	TX
		Lackland AFB	TX
		Portsmouth NH	VA
		Ft. Lewis	WA

Employing Excess MTF Capacity and Sustaining the MTF's Case Mix

The minimum-MTF case considers a substantial reduction in the size of the military system and, as a result, raises additional issues. An important issue is: To what degree would military hospitals need other than local, active-duty patients to fill their capacity in peacetime?

In FY92, the eleven hospitals in the military-care option admitted about 224,000 patients, while the six hospitals in the reception-and-referral option admitted over 135,000 patients. In each case, about 28 percent of the admissions were active-duty personnel—not a sufficient number to sustain the staffing of these hospitals. They would clearly require a significant number of other patients. While some would argue that the roughly 200,000 active-duty hospitalizations in 1992 would fill the military hospitals in the reception-and-referral option and nearly fill them in the military-care option, such an approach would lead to the wrong case mix for the physicians required in wartime and would involve tremendous costs of moving large numbers of military personnel around the United States. We therefore reject such an approach as inefficient and likely to generate excessive costs.

To provide workload and the right case mix, this case assumes that DoD's contracts with civilian health plans would require that they reimburse for services provided in MTFs and that their managed-care plans refer to the MTFs to fill capacity. Versions of both provisions already exist. Military hospitals are reimbursed by private insurance for military patients with such insurance and for nonmilitary patients, although collecting from the many private plans is

Table 11

Military Hospitals Converted to Clinics in the Minimum-MTF Case

Clinic	Year 92	97	Clinic	Year 92	97	Clinic	Year 92	97
Redstone Arsl, AL	C	C	Ft. Gordon, GA	C	C	Griffiss AFB, NY	C	
Ft. McClellan, AL	C	C	Ft. Benning, GA	C	C	Ft. Bragg, NC*	C	C
Ft. Rucker, AL	C	C	Ft. Stewart, GA	C	C	Seymour Jnsn, NC	C	C
Maxwell AFB, AL	C	C	Moody AFB, GA	C	C	Cmp Lejeune, NC*	C	C
Ft. Wainwright, AK	C	C	Robins AFB, GA	C	C	Cherry Point, NC	C	C
Elmendorf AFB, AK	C	C	Ft. Shafter, HI*	C	C	Grand Forks, ND	C	C
Adak NH, AK	C	C	Mountain Hme, ID	C	C	Minot AFB, ND	C	C
Ft. Huachuca, AZ	C	C	Chanute AFB, IL	C		Wright-Patt, OH	C	C
Luke AFB, AZ	C	C	Scott AFB, IL	C	C	Tinker AFB, OK	C	C
Davis Monthan, AZ	C	C	Great Lakes, IL	C	C	Altus AFB, OK	C	C
Little Rock, AR	C	C	Ft. Ben Hrrsn, IN	C		Ft. Sill, OK	C	C
Travis AFB, CA	C	C	Ft. Riley, KS	C	C	Newport NH, RI	C	C
Beale AFB, CA	C	C	Ft. Leavnwrth, KS	C	C	Shaw AFB, SC	C	C
McClellan AFB, CA	C	C	Ft. Campbell, KY*	C	C	Charlestn NH, SC	C	C
Castle AFB, CA	C		Ft. Knox, KY	C	C	Beaufort NH, SC	C	C
Vandenbrg AFB, CA	C	C	Barksdle AFB, LA	C	C	Ft. Jackson, SC	C	C
Edwards AFB, CA	C	C	Ft. Polk, LA	C	C	Ellswrth AFB, SD	C	C
March AFB, CA	C		Loring AFB, ME	C		Millingtn NH, TN	C	C
Presidio, CA	C		Andrews AFB, MD	C	C	Ft. Bliss, TX	C	C
Ft. Ord, CA	C		Bethesda NH, MD	C	C	Ft. Sam Hstn, TX	C	C
Camp Pendletn, CA	C	C	Patuxent Rvr, MD	C	C	Ft. Hood, TX*	C	C
Long Beach NH, CA	C		Ft. Meade, MD	C	C	Reese AFB, TX	C	C
Oakland NH, CA	C		Ft. Devens, MA	C		Dyess AFB, TX	C	C
Lemoore NH, CA	C	C	K.I. Sawyer, MI	C		Sheppard AFB, TX	C	C
29 Palms, CA	C	C	Keesler AFB, MS	C	C	Laughlin AFB, TX	C	C
Ft. Irwin, CA	C	C	Columbus AFB, MS	C	C	Bergstrm AFB, TX	C	
Fitzsmmns AMC, CO	C	C	Ft. Leonrd Wd, MO	C	C	Carswell AFB, TX	C	
Ft. Carson, CO	C	C	Whiteman AFB, MO	C	C	Corpus Chsti, TX	C	C
USAF Academy, CO	C	C	Offutt AFB, NE	C	C	Hill AFB, UT	C	C
Groton NH, CT	C	C	Nellis AFB, NV	C	C	Langley AFB, VA	C	C
Dover AFB, DE**	C	C	Ft. Monmouth, NJ	C	C	Ft. Eustis, VA	C	C
Pensacola NH, FL	C	C	McGuire AFB, NJ	C	C	Ft. Lee, VA	C	C
Jacksonville, FL*	C	C	Kirtland AFB, NM	C	C	Ft. Belvoir, VA	C	C
Orlando NH, FL	C		Holloman AFB, NM	C	C	Bremerton NH, WA	C	C
Eglin AFB, FL	C	C	Cannon AFB, NM	C	C	Oak Harbor, WA	C	C
Tyndall AFB,FL	C	C	West Point, NY	C	C	Fairchld AFB, WA	C	C
MacDill AFB, FL	C	C	Plattsburg, NY	C		FE Warrn AFB, WY	C	C
Patrick AFB, FL	C	C						

*These MTFs are clinics only in the "reception-and-referral" option.
**These MTFs are clinics only in the "military-care" option.

difficult. A requirement to refer patients to the MTFs when possible is included in current CRI contracts. Such an arrangement allows us to include the cost of any MTF care provided to non-active-duty beneficiaries in civilian plan rates.

The Military-Civilian Competition Case (#4)

The fourth case would offer most non-active-duty beneficiaries the choice of a military HMO plan based on the MTFs or one or more commercial health plans. All active-duty personnel would be enrolled in the military HMO if assigned to an MTF area; otherwise, they would receive care through small clinics as in the third case. MTFs would be responsible for all health care for beneficiaries who chose to enroll in the military plan, although some services would be provided by civilian providers at MTF expense. The MTFs' budgets for peacetime health care delivery would be based on a per-capita "payment" for each enrollee.

Non-active-duty beneficiaries who preferred civilian care would be offered one or more commercial plans (if possible, at least one HMO and one PPO and/or FFS plan). These beneficiaries would receive all of their care through the commercial plan they chose, and they would not be eligible for any care at the MTF. In areas where the military plan could not be offered, only commercial plans would be available.[14] All beneficiaries would receive health care only within the plan they chose, with no health care provided outside the enrolled plan.[15] CHAMPUS would be terminated.

We assumed the different plans in this case would have benefits (e.g., deductibles, copayments, coverages) similar to those of current plans:

- Military HMO: the benefits offered in CRI Prime (the HMO option),
- FFS plans: current CHAMPUS benefits,
- Civilian HMOs: the benefits offered in HMOs available through the Federal Employees Health Benefits Plan.

If military beneficiaries are ever given a direct choice between military and civilian health plans, premiums will be the most direct policy tool for ensuring sufficient enrollment in the military plan to fill MTF capacity. Therefore, in this case we varied the premium contribution beneficiaries would have to pay for these plans to see how differential premium costs might affect enrollment in the military HMO. We considered two premium structures: equal premiums for all

---

[14]Some beneficiaries in noncatchment areas, especially those living just beyond catchment-area boundaries, may prefer enrollment in an MTF HMO rather than one of the civilian options. Although the analysis could consider such a choice as a variant of this basic alternative design, it would affect costs only if there were a significant number of such beneficiaries and if the MTF plan were significantly more or less expensive than commercial plans.

[15]DoD could ensure that all active-duty dependents are covered by mandating a default enrollment choice for all eligible dependents; this requirement could be waived for those who offer proof of private insurance coverage. With national health reform, DoD might collect premium contributions from private employers and even contribute the premium for employer plans.

plans (either none or about 20 percent of the typical plan's cost) and premiums only for civilian plans (again, about 20 percent).

The per-capita cost of care in the military HMO would depend on the level of utilization by enrollees. As we described in Section 3, current utilization levels for military beneficiaries are high. Reorganizing the MTFs to operate like the most cost-effective civilian HMOs would lower inpatient utilization levels in particular. Alternatively, the military plans might require enrollees to pay a share of the costs of their care, forgoing the tight utilization controls associated with an HMO. To explore the cost implications of these different approaches, we estimated three sets of utilization rates for military HMO enrollees, based on: (1) current utilization by the military population, (2) civilian HMO utilization, and (3) utilization under cost-sharing arrangements.

For this case, the MTF hospitals will be as specified in Table 6 for case 1. All military clinics would remain open to treat active-duty personnel, but we have not assumed that they would offer the HMO plan. Conceivably, some of these clinics could operate an HMO by directly providing primary care and either arranging for more specialized services within the MTF system or contracting with civilian providers for such services as civilian IPAs do now. However, our data were not adequate for estimating utilization and costs for clinic-based HMOs.

A Comparison of the Four Analytic Cases

Tables 12 and 13 show the number of MTFs and the proportion of the population who are expected to live near them in 1997. Figures 13–15 map the hospital catchment areas and clinic service areas in 1997.[16]

The managed-care case (Figure 13) would serve a large fraction of military beneficiaries in the United States. Most active-duty personnel and their dependents would live in areas with a hospital (Table 13).[17] Just over one-half of retiree and survivor families would live near an MTF. The military-civilian competition case assumes that some military hospitals continue to operate, but

---

[16] These figures assume that all catchment areas reach out 40 miles, whereas in reality catchment areas are defined by ZIP codes and may have a smaller radius based on physical barriers (such as rivers and bays), state boundaries, and overlaps with other catchment areas. In cases of overlaps, ZIP-code assignments sometimes vary by service; for example, naval personnel in Washington, D.C., are assigned to Bethesda Naval Hospital, whereas Army personnel are assigned to Walter Reed Army Medical Center.

[17] The fractions would be even higher if we were to include areas with a military clinic in Table 13—94 percent for active-duty personnel and 89 percent for their dependents.

Table 12

Estimated Number of MTFs Under Each Case

Case	1992		1997	
	Hospitals	Clinics	Hospitals	Clinics
1. Managed care	117	74	101	86
2. Maximum MTF	118	72	108	72
3. Minimum MTF				
a) Reception/referral	6	128	6	118
b) Military care	11	123	11	113
4. Military-civilian competition	117	30	101	40

Table 13

Percentage of Military Beneficiaries in 1997 Catchment/Service Areas

Case	Active Duty	Active-Duty Dependents	Retirees and Dependents
1. Managed care	87%	80%	57%
2. Maximum MTF	89%	83%	64%
3. Minimum MTF			
a. Reception/referral	25%	—	—
b. Military care	41%	—	—
4. Military-civilian competition	87%	80%	57%

NOTE: Percentages are shown for active-duty personnel only for case 3 because other beneficiaries are enrolled in civilian health plans and would get care from MTFs only through contract with their civilian plan.

RANDMR407/1-13

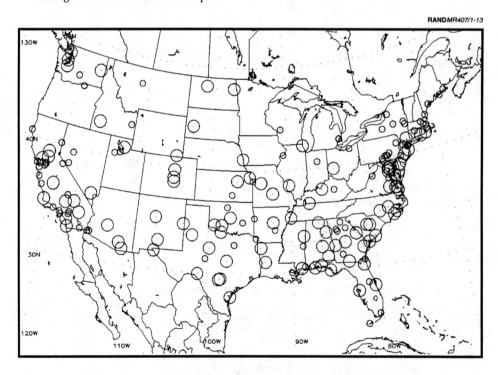

Figure 13—Locating 1997 MTFs for the Managed-Care and Military-Civilian Competition Cases

the clinics would serve only active-duty personnel. The MTFs in this case would cover essentially the same fraction of the active-duty population as the baseline case, but they would cover fewer non-active-duty beneficiaries. The maximum-MTF case (Figure 14) would have its greatest effect on the retired population and their dependents, raising the fraction who have access to a military hospital to almost two-thirds. The military hospitals retained in the minimum-MTF case (Figure 15) would serve only about 25 to 40 percent of active-duty personnel. However, with the added clinics the system would cover 90 percent in the United States (not shown)—only slightly less than the baseline managed-care case.

RAND*MR407/1-14*

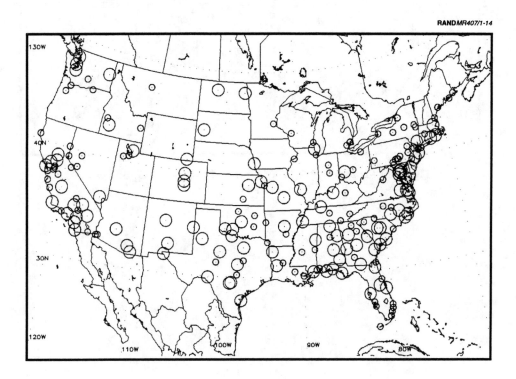

Figure 14—Locating 1997 MTFs for the Maximum-MTF Case

RAND*MR407/1-15*

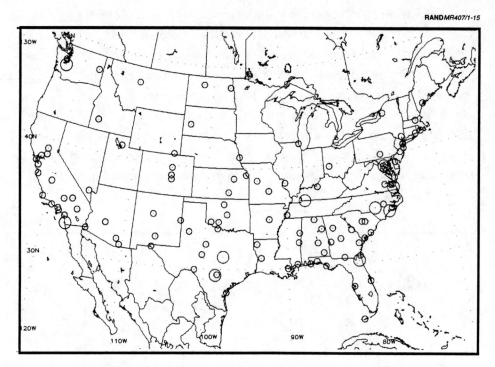

**Figure 15—Locating 1997 MTFs for the Military-Care Option of the
Minimum-MTF Case**

5. The Effects of Changes in the MHSS on Health Care Demand

Military beneficiaries' demand for health care is determined by numerous factors (as we discussed in Section 3), including:

- Personal characteristics,

- Family characteristics,

- Local (military and civilian) health-system characteristics, and

- Health-plan characteristics.

Although these factors are the same as those that shape health care demand in nonmilitary populations, the precise effects of each factor may differ in the two populations. Within the military population, there would also appear to be demand differences across the services that are not explained by these factors.

To illustrate effects on military health care utilization, Table 14 shows how demand for health care on the part of retirees and their dependents (under age 65) varies with two of these factors—health status and MTF capacity. Health status is measured by the number of reported health conditions (0–2 versus 3 or more), and MTFs are categorized according to whether their operating beds per 1,000 beneficiaries are above or below the median for all MTFs. The table shows that MTF utilization is higher in areas with more MTF capacity in relation to the beneficiary population, whereas civilian utilization is lower. At the same time, utilization in both sectors is higher for less healthy beneficiaries. These data are based on the beneficiary sample surveyed for the study and are weighted to reflect the population of retirees and dependents under age 65 in the United States.

Our task was to predict the effects of changing a subset of these factors—e.g., the size of the MTF system, nationwide implementation of managed care, or offering a choice of current health plans and commercial plans—on health care utilization and civilian health care costs. To do this, we had to be able to estimate the effects of changing these factors while holding all other factors constant. As an example, consider the prediction of utilization and cost in a system with a larger MTF capacity. To simulate only the effect of expanding MTFs, we would need to hold constant health status and other factors that influence demand. To do so, we

Table 14

**Average Health Care Utilization by Health Status and MTF
Capacity, Retirees and Dependents Under Age 65 Living in U.S.**

	Noncatchment areas	Catchment Areas: MTF Beds/1,000 Beneficiaries	
		1.34 & Under	Over 1.34
Healthier beneficiaries			
MTF visits	0.74	1.10	1.47
Civilian visits	1.40	1.05	0.79
Total MHSS visits	2.14	2.15	2.26
MTF hospital days	.007	.098	.295
Civilian hospital days	.083	.049	.070
Total MHSS days	.090	.147	.365
Less healthy beneficiaries			
MTF visits	0.82	2.62	3.21
Civilian visits	3.54	2.55	1.55
Total MHSS visits	4.36	5.17	4.76
MTF hospital days	.109	.232	.627
Civilian hospital days	.302	.185	.227
Total hospital days	.411	.417	.854

could construct average utilization rates by demand factor and beneficiary group, but sorting out all the important factors would require a very large table; for many of the cells, there would be insufficient data to measure utilization rates. Instead, we applied statistical methods to these data to accomplish the same purpose.

Methodology

Although the analytic methods we used were similar for all the analytic cases studied, such methods did differ depending on whether a given case was structured like the current MHSS—with MTFs and civilian health care financed by CHAMPUS (cases 1 and 2), or whether it incorporated commercial health plans as well (cases 3 and 4). This section first describes the methods we used to study cases based on the current system and then summarizes the results.[1] Our analysis involved the following four steps:

1. Structuring the analysis through the determination of the components of demand and the beneficiary groups to be analyzed;

---

[1] Our final report will include a second section that focuses on alternatives that encompass commercial health plans.

2. Development of measures of demand (utilization and cost) and of the factors that affect demand;

3. Estimation of demand equations for each demand component and beneficiary group that describe the independent effects of individual, family, and health-system factors on utilization and civilian care costs in the MHSS; and

4. Use of the equations derived in step 3 to predict utilization and civilian care costs in the analytic cases that represent alternative military health care systems.

The study's beneficiary survey served as the principal data source for this analysis. As described earlier, the survey was fielded during the winter and spring of 1992–1993 and provided information on about 16,000 active-duty, retiree, and survivor households eligible for military health care.[2] We augmented the survey data with information from CHAMPUS claims, the MEPRS and biometrics data systems, and the 1990 Area Resource File.

Structuring the Demand Analysis

The two "sectors" of the current MHSS—the MTFs and CHAMPUS—differ in the range of health services they cover, in the extent of beneficiary access, and in their cost both to beneficiaries and to DoD. Within each sector, beneficiaries may obtain outpatient care, measured in visits, as well as inpatient care, measured in hospital admissions. We further decomposed each of these four components of utilization—MTF visits, MTF admissions, CHAMPUS visits, and CHAMPUS admissions—into two components: the probability of having some utilization, and the level of utilization only for those beneficiaries who had some utilization. This decomposition of health care utilization into probability and level of use for outpatient and inpatient care is frequently used by health researchers. We similarly structured our analysis of CHAMPUS costs[3] in two parts: the probability of incurring nonzero CHAMPUS costs and the level of costs for those who had some costs. This structure resulted in ten components of demand.

As Table 15 shows, we conducted a full analysis for only eight of the ten components thus derived. Since very few beneficiaries are admitted to the hospital more than once per year, and since other studies have shown that the level of inpatient utilization is relatively unresponsive to demand factors, we did

---

[2]This excludes overseas populations, single active-duty personnel, and Reserve retirees. See Lurie et al. (1994) for more information regarding this survey.

[3]MTF costs are estimated by IDA in a separate report (Goldberg et al., 1994).

Table 15

Components of Demand Analyzed

MHSS Sector		Components
MTF	Utilization:	1. Probability of using any outpatient care
		2. For outpatient users only, number of visits
		3. Probability of using any inpatient care
CHAMPUS	Utilization:	1. Probability of using any outpatient care
		2. For outpatient users only, number of visits
		3. Probability of using any inpatient care
	Costs:	4. Probability of incurring any costs
		5. For those with costs, the level of costs

not attempt to analyze the number of admissions either in the MTFs or in CHAMPUS. Instead, this component of demand was held constant across the cases studied.

The demand analysis focused on active-duty dependents, retirees and their dependents, and survivors and their dependents living in the United States.[4] We assumed that because of the readiness mission, active-duty personnel would receive the same health care services they now obtain in all cases. Total active-duty utilization therefore varies only with the number of active-duty personnel. With the data available, an analysis of MTF utilization by beneficiaries living overseas, DoD's civilian employees, retired Reserve personnel, or other populations was not possible; hence the per-capita utilization rates of such personnel were also held constant across the cases.

The beneficiaries whom we studied were grouped as shown in Table 16 to accommodate differences in the structure of their health care demand. The analysis separated beneficiaries who live in MTF catchment areas from those in noncatchment areas because of the obvious difference in their access to MTF services. Further groupings differed for the MTF and CHAMPUS analyses. For MTF utilization, which we measured for individual beneficiaries, we grouped the catchment-area population according to CHAMPUS eligibility and age. Owing to their small sample size, the non-catchment-area population was studied in one group. In all instances, we assigned survey respondents to these groups according to the home ZIP code they reported in the survey rather than according to the location reported by DEERS.

---

[4]The 50 states and the District of Columbia.

Table 16

Population Groups Whose Demand Was Analyzed Separately

MTF Utilization
(unit of observation is the individual beneficiary)

	CHAMPUS Adult Eligibles	Children	Medicare Eligibles
Catchment Areas	I	II	III
Noncatchment Areas		IV	

CHAMPUS Utilization and Costs
(unit of observation is the family)

	Active-Duty Families	Retired Families
Catchment Areas	I	II
Noncatchment Areas	III	IV

For CHAMPUS utilization and cost, we had data for entire families, not just individuals. Our use of family-level data facilitated the analysis of civilian health costs in particular. Since costs are highly variable, they are difficult to predict with any precision; summing costs across family members allowed us to effectively increase the number of people being studied and decrease the proportion of the sample with zero costs. In addition, it was easier for us to match claims records to families, which is done by sponsor social security number, than to individuals, which also requires a series of difficult matches on sometimes inaccurate birthdate and sex information.[5]

The population of families with CHAMPUS-eligible members was grouped as shown in Table 16. Owing to the differences in CHAMPUS cost-sharing requirements, separate analyses were conducted for active-duty and retiree families in catchment areas; the sample in noncatchment areas was too small to separate the two family groups.

---

[5]Family-level analysis was not possible for MTF utilization because the survey asked for utilization by source of care only for a single family member.

Defining Measures of Demand and Factors Affecting Demand

Utilization and cost data were obtained from the self-reported survey data on MTF outpatient utilization and FY92 MTF inpatient records and CHAMPUS claims records for the survey respondents. We used a CHAMPUS hospital-episode file created by the Army's Directorate of Health Care Studies and Analyses, but we processed the outpatient claims ourselves. We defined a CHAMPUS outpatient visit for each same-patient/same-provider/same-day combination if the procedure codes indicated that an encounter with a provider had occurred. If only ancillary services had been provided, we did not define a visit. We summed costs from all hospital and professional inpatient claims and outpatient claims for each family and random family member.

Table 17 lists the variables that were included in the demand regressions as determinants of utilization and costs. Not all variables were included in every equation; for example, the MTF variables were not included in regressions for people living in noncatchment areas. In addition, some variables were deleted from some or all of the equations because they did not significantly affect demand. Education has elsewhere been shown to affect demand in other populations but did not do so in this population; the variable for officers (as opposed to enlisted personnel) includes the effects of education as well as other military-specific effects.

We did not include variables measuring premiums, deductibles, and copayment levels because there is little variation in cost sharing currently in the MHSS. We did identify those individuals who were subject to different cost-sharing arrangements through CRI and CAM. We did not include a variable indicating those with other insurance coverage because the decision to take such coverage is influenced by health care utilization. Instead, we included a variable indicating those who might have access to other insurance because someone in their family is employed on a full-time basis. Finally, the survey did not include a question about distance or travel time to the nearest MTF—an important factor in demand for care in the MTFs and CHAMPUS.

We defined many of these variables in an obvious manner from the survey information. However, some were obtained from other data sources or require additional explanation.

Table 17

Individual, Family, and Health Care Characteristics Included in Demand Regressions

Type	Variable
Individual characteristics[a]	Age
	Sex
	Number of reported health conditions
Family characteristics	Age of spouse or (if no spouse) sponsor[b]
	Sponsor is an officer
	Sponsor not affiliated with military service that operates MTF (catchment areas only)
	Sponsor (retired only) or spouse is employed full time
	Income
	Number of family members
	Enrolled in CRI Prime
	Living in CRI area but not enrolled
	Enrolled in Air Force CAM plan
	Living in Air Force CAM area but not enrolled
	Enrolled in Navy CAM plan
	Living in Navy CAM area but not enrolled
	Minimum health status for any family member[b]
MTF characteristics	Military service
	Operating beds per 1,000 military population in catchment area
	Clinical staff per operating bed
	County has military clinic that provides outpatient care (>1 visit per year) to non-active-duty beneficiaries[c]
Civilian health characteristics	Beds per 1,000 total population in county
	Physicians (active) per 1,000 total population in county

[a]MTF regressions only.
[b]CHAMPUS regressions only.
[c]Noncatchment areas only.

Individual Characteristics

We defined a number of age variables that capture the relationship between age and health care use shown in Figure 3. For all groups, we included a variable for age squared as well as for age. For regressions that included active-duty spouses, we also included a variable to indicate women of child-bearing age (18 to 34) because their use is high during these years. When we combined children and adults—e.g., in noncatchment areas—we defined different age variables for the two groups. We experimented with several ways of representing information on health conditions; we used a simple count of the number of conditions reported because it was effective in explaining demand and because it allowed us to keep the variable list short—an advantage for statistical reasons.

Family Characteristics

With the exception of the CRI and CAM enrollment variables, the family variables are straightforward. The survey question combined CRI's CHAMPUS Prime (the enrollment plan) and CHAMPUS Extra (the optional PPO) options in the same answer, but we wanted to identify just those who had enrolled in Prime. We also found that respondents who lived in CAM areas sometimes reported that they were enrolled in Prime, which happens to be the name of the Navy's enrollment plan as well. In addition, we modified the survey data to make them more consistent. If the ZIP code reported by the respondent was in a CRI area, we considered the family to be enrolled if (s)he reported that the family used CHAMPUS Prime/Extra. We included all of these people because doing so gave us enrollment rates that were very close to those reported by the CRI contractor at the time of the survey. If the ZIP code was in a CAM area, we considered the family to be enrolled if they reported use of either CHAMPUS Prime/Extra or the appropriate CAM program. As for CRI, the enrollment rates we obtained in this way were consistent with other information on enrollment.

MTF Characteristics

We used the MTF data available through the DMIS data systems with some modifications. Since the recorded number of operating beds was out of date for many MTFs, we replaced it with information collected more recently by Health Affairs. We also corrected the DEERS catchment-area population counts for the more important discrepancies described in Section 3. We used MEPRS MTF staffing data for FY92, combining the data for hospitals and clinics in the same catchment area and, where possible, deleting staffing in satellite clinics located outside catchment areas. We also combined several catchment areas that substantially overlapped; these included areas in and near the District of Columbia, San Antonio, and Colorado Springs.

For the noncatchment population, we determined whether areas were served by a military clinic by matching respondents to counties using reported ZIP codes and by identifying those counties with a military clinic. We deleted clinics that reported under one visit per non-active-duty beneficiary in the FY92 biometrics reports. We also explored the possibility of further differentiating areas with clinics that provide a higher level of service to these beneficiaries, but our sample proved too small to make this feasible.

Civilian Health Characteristics

Again using ZIP-code information, we matched respondents to county data on hospital beds, physicians, and population in the 1990 Area Resource File—the most recent data available in a single source.

Estimating Demand Equations

The structure developed in step 1 required that we estimate twelve MTF utilization equations (three components of demand for each of four groups of individual beneficiaries), twelve CHAMPUS utilization equations (the same three components for each of four groups of families), and eight CHAMPUS cost equations (two components of cost for the four family groups). Each equation quantifies the relationship between a component of utilization or cost and the factors—the independent variables in the equation—that determine that particular component. The equations are estimated separately using standard multiple regression techniques, as described more fully in Appendix C.

Predicting Utilization and Costs for the Analytic Cases

Utilization and costs for the analytic cases were generated from the demand equations. The first step lay in determining which demand factors would change in each case and how they would change. (The manner in which this was done for the expanded-MTF case is described below.) Then, for each individual or family in the survey sample, we substituted revised values for the variables that measure the factors that change. The updated variables were entered into the demand equations to obtain a prediction for each individual or family for each component of demand and, subsequently, for the utilization and cost measures of interest: MTF visits, MTF admissions, CHAMPUS visits, CHAMPUS admissions, and CHAMPUS costs. We estimated per-capita utilization and costs for the population by averaging the predictions for individuals (MTF) and families (CHAMPUS), weighting the survey sample so that it reflected the DoD population as a whole, not just survey participants. Finally, we estimated total utilization and costs by multiplying the per-capita averages for the population by the total number of individuals and families in the population.

The base case used in our analysis is the current military system with managed care—specifically a CRI-type program—in all catchment areas. Since 1988, the military health care system has adopted a number of reforms, the most important of which is managed care. Only a part of the system now has managed-care programs, but DoD is moving rapidly to expand CRI-like programs nationwide.

Since information about the expansion of managed care to noncatchment areas is limited, we did not attempt to estimate utilization and costs with managed care in these areas. As part of the regression analysis, the change in demand associated with managed care was estimated from the current CRI programs. However, since DoD plans some changes in future CRI programs, and to the extent that there is some uncertainty regarding our estimates of the effects even of the current CRI program, we also investigated the sensitivity of our results to the type of program we chose to simulate.

Although we sought to replicate as closely as possible DoD's immediate plans, our primary purpose in simulating nationwide implementation of managed care for case 1 (the "baseline" system) was technical: to keep other conditions the same when predicting the effects of the changes envisioned in case 2. Unless we simulated proportional increases in MTF capacity in all areas, we might otherwise "grow" managed-care areas more or less than "standard" areas and mistakenly attribute the results entirely to changes in case 2. Instead of CRI, we could have simulated a baseline case without managed care in any area. We chose to base case 1 on CRI because it is most similar to current DoD plans for the future. In addition, CRI has been tested in numerous catchment areas (instead of two currently for CAM), so our estimates of program effects are less likely to be affected by local circumstances unrelated to managed care.

The specific procedure used to predict utilization and costs for the analytic cases depended on the specific changes envisioned in each case. The following describes the procedures used for the expanded-MTF case. Like the base case, the expanded-MTF case incorporates managed care. In addition, as described in Section 4, it supposes an expanded version of the FY92 MTF system that included the following:

- A military hospital in Atlanta, Georgia;
- Expanded physical capacity (as measured by the number of operating beds) at 16 existing military hospitals; and
- Increased staffing levels at most hospitals.

Prediction of utilization and costs for this case required only limited changes in the variables in the demand equations. For example, we reassigned the beneficiaries in our sample who live in the Atlanta catchment area from the non-catchment-area group to the catchment-area group and assumed that they would have access to an MTF with operating beds and staff appropriate to the Atlanta catchment-area military population. Their utilization and costs are then predicted using catchment-area demand equations. Beneficiaries already living in a catchment area stay in the same population group, and their utilization and costs are predicted using the demand equations for that group, but the variables that describe their MTF might change.

In both the baseline and expanded-MTF cases, we needed to incorporate the effects of expanding CRI to all catchment areas. We assumed that each active-duty dependent has a 35 percent probability, and each retiree and dependent a 26 percent probability, of enrolling in the managed-care plan; these are the enrollment rates reported in the survey for CRI populations. Each person's utilization (or cost) is predicted to be a weighted average of utilization if enrolled and utilization if not enrolled, with the enrollment probability used as the weight.

The final prediction step is a series of adjustments to the predictions. For MTF utilization, this step adds the predicted utilization for the population groups studied to the current utilization for the groups held constant or not studied— e.g., active-duty personnel and overseas beneficiaries. It also adjusts the predicted visits and admissions, derived from the survey data, to make them compatible with the data that are reported in MEPRS, and it allocates the utilization to the individual MTFs. The survey-MEPRS adjustment is necessary because IDA uses MEPRS data in estimating the cost functions that are applied to our utilization estimates to obtain MTF costs. Appendix D provides more information about these MTF utilization adjustments. CHAMPUS utilization is not adjusted, but CHAMPUS costs are inflated both to include claims processing and other overhead costs and to correct for any incompleteness.[6]

Effects of Demand Factors: Summary of Regression Results

To aid in understanding the utilization projections for the different analytic cases, we summarize here the effects of the variables listed above on past utilization, as reflected in the demand equations. Tables 18 to 20 indicate whether each factor increases or decreases each component of demand. The sample sizes, estimated coefficients, and standard errors for the regressions are reported in Appendix C.

---

[6]We estimated completed costs from the CHAMPUS Health Care Summary Report using the completion factor calculated by CHAMPUS for that report. We then multiplied our cost estimates by the percentage our estimate of current CHAMPUS costs differed from the adjusted CHAMPUS figure. Like the CHAMPUS reports, our data were incomplete.

Table 18

Summary of Regression Results for MTF Outpatient Visits and Hospital Admissions

Variable	Catchment adults			Catchment children			Catchment Medicare			Noncatchment (all)		
	Visits		Adm.	Visits		Adm.	Visits		Adm.	Visits		Adm.
	>0	no.	>0	>0	no.	>0	>0	no.	>0	>0	no.	>0
Age	+	(+)	(-)	(-)	-	-	-		(+)	(+)		(-)
Age squared	-	(+)	(+)	(-)	-	+		+		-	(+)	+
Retiree/dependent	-	-	(-)	(+)	+	-					+	(+)
Medicare eligible										+		+
Female retiree/dep.	+	+	-	+		+	(-)		-	+		
Female age 18–34	+	+	(+)	+	+		(+)	+			+	(+)
Health status	(+)	+	+	-	-	+	+	+	+	+	-	+
Officer	-	(-)	-	(+)	(+)	(-)	(+)	(-)	(-)	(-)		(-)
Not MTF's service	-	-	-	-	+	+	-	(+)	(+)			(+)
Employed full time	(+)			+	+	-				-		+
Income	-	(-)	(-)	(-)	(-)	(+)	(-)	+	+	(-)	(-)	(-)
Income—retired	+	+	(-)	+	+	(+)	-	+	-	-	-	(+)
No. in family		+	(+)		+							-
CRI/enrolled												
AD dependents	(-)	(-)	(-)	(-)	(-)	(+)	(+)				(+)	(-)
Retirees/others	(+)	(+)	(+)	(+)	(+)	(+)	+				(+)	(+)
AF CAM/enrolled												
AD dependents	(-)	(+)	(-)	(-)	(-)	(-)						(-)
Retirees/others	(-)	(+)		(+)	(-)							
Navy CAM/enrolled												
AD dependents	(+)	(-)		(-)	(-)	(-)						(-)
Retirees/others	(+)	(-)	(+)	(+)	(+)							(+)
Army vs. AF MTF	-	+	(+)	-	-	-	(+)	(-)	-	+	-	(+)
Navy vs. AF MTF	-	(+)	(+)	-	-	-	+	(+)	+	-	(+)	(-)
MTF beds/1000	+	+	(+)	+	+	+	(-)	(+)	(+)			(-)
MTF MDs/bed	+	+		+	+					+		
Mil. clinic										+	-	(-)

NOTE: ( ) indicates that the coefficient is not statistically significant at the .05 level. Variables with no sign were not included in the regression.

Table 19

Summary of Regression Results for CHAMPUS Outpatient Visits and Hospital Admissions

Variable	Catchment-area active duty Outpatient >0	Outpatient no.	Adm. >0	Catchment-area retired Outpatient >0	Outpatient no.	Adm. >0	Noncatchment areas (all) Outpatient >0	Outpatient no.	Adm. >0
Spouse/sponsor age	+	(+)	(-)	+	(-)	(+)	(+)	(+)	(+)
Sp. age squared	-	(-)	(+)	(-)	(+)	(-)	(-)	(+)	(-)
Fam. health status	+	+	+	+	+	+	+	+	+
Officer	+	+	(+)	+	+	(-)	+	+	+
Employed full time	(+)	+	-	-	(+)	(-)	+	(-)	(+)
Income	+	+	(-)	+	+	(+)	+	(+)	(+)
No. in family	+	+	+	+	(+)	+	+	+	(+)
CRI/enrolled	+	+	+	+	+	+			
CRI/standard	-	+	-	-	(+)	(-)			
AF CAM/enrolled	(+)	(+)	(-)	+	(-)	(+)			
AF CAM/standard	(-)	(-)	(-)	(+)	(+)	(-)			
Navy CAM/enrolled	+	(+)	(-)	(+)	(+)	(+)			
Navy CAM/standard	(+)	(-)	+	(-)	(-)	(-)			
Army vs. AF MTF	(-)	(+)	(+)	+	+	(+)			
Navy vs. AF MTF	+	+	+	-	-	(+)			
MTF beds/1000	-	-	-	-	-				
MTF MDs/bed	-	-	-		(-)	-			
Mil. clinic area				+	(+)	(-)			
Civ. beds/1000	(+)	(-)	(+)	-	(-)	(+)	(+)	(-)	(-)
Civ. MDs/1000	-	+	(+)	-		(-)	-	+	-

NOTE: ( ) indicates that the coefficient is not statistically significant at the .05 level. Variables with no sign were not included in the regression.

Table 20

Summary of Regression Results for CHAMPUS Costs (paid by DoD)

Variable	Catchment-area active duty		Catchment-area retired		Noncatchment areas (all)	
	>$0	$ Amount	>$0	$ Amount	>$0	$ Amount
Spouse/sponsor age	+	(+)	+	−	(+)	+
Sp. age squared	(−)	(−)	(−)	+	(−)	−
Child < 1 year old	+	+	(+)	(−)	−	(+)
Retired					+	+
Fam. health status	+	+	+	+	+	+
Officer	+	(+)	(+)	+	+	+
Employed full time	(−)	−	(−)	(−)	−	−
Income	(−)	(−)	+	(−)	(+)	(−)
Income—ret.					+	+
No. in family	+	+	+	+		
CRI/enrolled	+	+	+	+		
CRI/standard	−	(+)	−	+		
AF CAM/enrolled	(+)	(+)	+	(−)		
AF CAM/standard	−	(+)	(−)	(+)		
Navy CAM/enrolled	+	(−)	(−)	(−)		
Navy CAM/standard	(−)	(+)	(+)	(+)		
Army vs. AF MTF	(−)	(−)	+	+		
Navy vs. AF MTF	(−)	(−)	(−)	(−)		
MTF beds/1000	−	−	(−)	(−)		
MTF MDs/bed		−	(−)	(+)	(+)	
Mil. clinic area	(+)	(+)	+	(+)	(+)	
Civ. beds/1000			−	(−)	−	(+)
Civ. MDs/1000	−	(+)				(+)

NOTE: ( ) indicates that the coefficient is not statistically significant at the .05 level. Variables with no sign were not included in the regression.

The estimated coefficients for age generally mirror the patterns seen in Figure 3. Poor health status is strongly and positively associated with higher utilization and costs. Members of the families of officers and sponsors from the same military service that operates the MTF typically are more likely to seek care; however, the higher propensity of officers' families to use MTF care is not statistically significant for most groups. As expected, those in a family with a full-time civilian worker are less likely to receive their care from MTFs, but that does not necessarily apply to CHAMPUS. Family income has no consistent relationship to demand, although higher-income families are more likely to use CHAMPUS.

Most measures of the propensity to use MTFs are lower for Army MTFs and almost all are lower for Navy MTFs than for Air Force MTFs. The managed-care programs (CRI and CAM) have no significant effect on MTF utilization, but enrollees use more CHAMPUS outpatient care. Inpatient CHAMPUS utilization seems to be lower for nonenrollees. MTF demand increases with MTF capacity, as measured by beds and clinical staffing per thousand beneficiaries in the area. By contrast, CHAMPUS demand decreases with capacity, suggesting that the two are substitutes. In noncatchment areas, access to a military clinic increases the propensity to use MTF outpatient care but does not decrease CHAMPUS outpatient use. The CHAMPUS cost results generally follow from the utilization results.

Predicted Demand in Baseline and Expanded MTF Cases (1 & 2)

Tables 21 to 25 summarize our predictions of utilization in the MTFs and CHAMPUS, and of CHAMPUS costs, for cases 1 and 2. As described in Section 4, case 1 is the current system with a nationwide managed-care program based on CRI. Case 2 is the same managed-care program with expanded MTF capacity. The outpatient utilization tables (Tables 21 and 23) show the predicted per-person visit rate for MTF services and the per-family rate for CHAMPUS services for cases 1 and 2 in the first two columns. The other four columns show predicted values for the two components of the visit rate: the probability of having any visits and the number of visits conditional on being a user. The inpatient utilization tables (Tables 22 and 24) show only the probability that a person or family has any hospital care.

MTF Utilization

Although overall utilization rates differ somewhat, the differences in utilization between the baseline and expanded-MTF cases are the same in 1992 and 1997.[7] For beneficiaries living in catchment areas in either year, we predict an increase of approximately 15 percent in MTF outpatient-service use by non-active-duty personnel with the added MTF capacity and higher staffing levels in case 2 (Table 21).[8] Sixty percent of the outpatient increase represents additional users and 40 percent higher levels of use. Many of the added visits are for CHAMPUS-eligible retirees and dependents. These beneficiaries have a lower priority for MTF care than do active-duty dependents, so it is not surprising that they benefit most when MTF capacity expands. It is surprising, however, that Medicare-eligible retirees and dependents do not show the same increase as the younger retired group. It may be that their utilization is constrained more by the lack of resources appropriate to treat the elderly in the many small military hospitals than by access to the services the MTFs can provide.

Table 21

MTF Outpatient Demand in Baseline and Expanded Cases (1 & 2) (FY 1992 and 1997 MTFs and populations)

Beneficiary Category	Visits/Person		Probability of Use		Visits/User	
	Baseline (1)	Expanded MTF (2)	Baseline (1)	Expanded MTF (2)	Baseline (1)	Expanded MTF (2)
1992						
Catchment areas	2.35	2.70	0.57	0.62	4.11	4.36
AD dependents	2.84	3.09	0.70	0.73	4.04	4.23
Retirees & deps.	1.95	2.50	0.47	0.56	4.05	4.44
Medicare	1.96	2.06	0.42	0.43	4.69	4.75
Other areas	0.97	0.97	0.24	0.24	4.00	4.01
All areas	1.95	2.22	0.47	0.51	4.10	4.31
1997						
Catchment areas	2.39	2.75	0.57	0.62	4.17	4.42
AD dependents	2.90	3.17	0.71	0.75	4.07	4.20
Retirees & deps.	2.08	2.63	0.49	0.58	4.17	4.38
Medicare	1.87	2.00	0.40	0.43	4.60	4.84
Other areas	0.93	0.93	0.23	0.23	4.08	4.09
All areas	1.84	2.10	0.44	0.48	4.15	4.36

---

[7]For the baseline case, average use for all beneficiaries will be lower in 1997, primarily because a larger fraction of beneficiaries will be living in noncatchment areas.

[8]Recall that the survey truncated the visits data at 10. The figures we report in these tables do not correct for this truncation.

We found only minor differences in MTF utilization between standard and either CRI or CAM areas, so these results would not change appreciably if we substituted the standard program or CAM for CRI in these two cases. We estimate, for example, that MTF outpatient utilization with CRI is under 1 percent higher than without CRI for CHAMPUS beneficiaries in catchment areas. The CRI evaluation also found a small increase in MTF outpatient utilization (just over 2 percent) two years into the program after controlling for preprogram differences in utilization between CRI and other areas (Hosek et al., 1993).

The overall increase in the proportion of catchment-area beneficiaries who use the MTFs' inpatient services in case 2—17 percent (Table 22)—is comparable to the outpatient increase of 15 percent. Here the difference is larger for active-duty dependents; the regression results show that inpatient utilization by adult retiree family members is more responsive to MTF capacity than that of adult active-duty family members, but the opposite is the case for the retirees' children.

As we discussed earlier, we considered a version of case 2 that would add 41 outpatient clinics as well as add one or more hospitals and expanded the hospitals' staffing. The regression analysis showed that MTF inpatient utilization actually declines when military outpatient clinics are added. MTF outpatient utilization increases by perhaps 10 percent; more people obtain MTF care, but

Table 22

**MTF Inpatient Demand in Baseline and Expanded Cases
(1 & 2) (FY 1992 and 1997 MTFs and populations)**

| | Probability of Hospital Use | |
| | Baseline | Expanded |
Beneficiary Category	(1)	MTF (2)
1992		
Catchment areas	0.062	0.075
AD dependents	0.086	0.104
Retirees & deps.	0.036	0.045
Medicare	0.062	0.074
Other areas	0.016	0.016
All areas	0.049	0.059
1997		
Catchment areas	0.063	0.077
AD dependents	0.091	0.110
Retirees & deps.	0.038	0.047
Medicare	0.058	0.071
Other areas	0.014	0.014
All areas	0.045	0.055

users have fewer MTF visits. As Table 23 shows, the MTF outpatient increase is complemented by a slight increase in non-catchment-area CHAMPUS outpatient utilization. These results suggest that beneficiaries in areas without a clinic may try to get their referral care in the MTFs but that beneficiaries who use outlying military clinics may be more likely to be referred to the local civilian community. We urge that caution be exercised in interpreting the predictions for noncatchment areas, however, because they are based on a small sample, and some uncertainty remains about the actual location of active-duty families in particular. It is also possible that people who live near a military clinic and people who live away from any MTF differ in other ways not captured in the regressions, and that these differences are engendering the utilization patterns we observe. For these reasons, we did not include the added clinics in the final version of case 2.

CHAMPUS Utilization

As expected, we project that beneficiary families living in catchment areas would decrease their CHAMPUS utilization if MTF capacity were expanded as envisioned in case 2. The results for 1992 and 1997 are very similar. We saw above that retirees and their dependents especially would use more MTF outpatient services, and Table 23 shows that they would also have the largest decrease in CHAMPUS outpatient use. CHAMPUS inpatient utilization also decreases in case 2—by about the same fraction for both catchment-area groups

Table 23

CHAMPUS Outpatient Demand in Baseline and Expanded Cases (1 & 2)
(FY 1992 and 1997 MTFs and populations)

Beneficiary Category	Visits/Family Baseline (1)	Visits/Family Expanded MTF (2)	Probability of Use Baseline (1)	Probability of Use Expanded MTF (2)	Visits/User Family Baseline (1)	Visits/User Family Expanded MTF (2)
			1992			
Catchment areas	4.05	3.48	0.39	0.36	10.35	9.73
Active duty	3.72	3.31	0.39	0.36	9.66	9.21
Retired < age 65	4.40	3.66	0.40	0.35	10.98	10.20
Other areas	5.83	5.81	0.52	0.52	11.10	11.08
All areas	4.54	4.11	0.43	0.40	10.61	10.18
			1997			
Catchment areas	3.79	3.27	0.38	0.35	9.96	9.41
AD dependents	3.58	3.14	0.38	0.35	9.51	9.08
Retirees & deps.	4.21	3.50	0.39	0.35	1.73	9.96
Other areas	5.84	5.79	0.53	0.53	11.02	10.93
All areas	4.42	4.00	0.43	0.40	10.37	9.97

(Table 24). Especially for active-duty dependents, the decrease in outpatient use is smaller than the decrease in inpatient use.

To estimate how total military-system utilization (MTF and CHAMPUS) in catchment areas would change with MTF expansion, we need to convert the per-family visit rates that we estimated for CHAMPUS to per-person rates. The average active-duty family has 2.59 CHAMPUS-eligible members, and the average non-Medicare retired family has 2.37 members. In catchment areas, then, the decrease in CHAMPUS use is 0.16 visit per active-duty dependent and 0.31 visit per retired family member—64 percent and 56 percent, respectively, of the increase in MTF visits.[9] With CHAMPUS outpatient use decreasing less than MTF use increases, we conclude that total demand for outpatient services by CHAMPUS eligibles increases as MTF capacity expands.

DoD defines the ratio of the change in MTF utilization to CHAMPUS utilization when MTF capacity is increased as the "tradeoff factor." Previous estimates of this factor were derived from aggregate MTF and CHAMPUS data and were for

Table 24

**CHAMPUS Inpatient Demand in Baseline and
Expanded Cases (1 & 2)
(FY 1992 and 1997 MTFs and Populations)**

Beneficiary Category	Probability of Use	
	Baseline (1)	Expanded MTF (2)
1992		
Catchment areas	0.038	0.031
AD dependents	0.042	0.034
Retirees & deps.	0.034	0.027
Other areas	0.076	0.076
All areas	0.048	0.043
1997		
Catchment areas	0.036	0.029
AD dependents	0.038	0.030
Retirees & deps.	0.033	0.026
Other areas	0.080	0.081
All areas	0.050	0.044

---

[9]Both our MTF and CHAMPUS visit estimates are subject to some error. As discussed in Section 3, the MTF data are subject to recall error and are therefore underestimated. CHAMPUS claims may be submitted for some time after the date of service; the data we received should be over 90 percent complete. With accurate data, we might expect that the decrease in CHAMPUS would be a somewhat smaller fraction of the increase in the MTFs. Therefore, the tradeoff factor should be higher with more accurate data.

64

all beneficiaries. Using these beneficiary-level data, we can estimate the tradeoff factor just for CHAMPUS-eligible beneficiaries living in catchment areas. Taking ratios of the estimated increase in MTF visits to the decrease in CHAMPUS visits as we move from case 1 to case 2, we calculate tradeoff factors of 1.56 for active-duty dependents and 1.79 for retirees, survivors, and their dependents. The tradeoff factor for the two combined is 1.67. Inclusion of other beneficiaries, such as those covered by Medicare for civilian care, would increase the tradeoff factor because there is no decrease in CHAMPUS to offset their increased MTF use.[10]

To calculate the tradeoff factor for inpatient services, we first multiply the probabilities in Tables 22 and 24 by the number of hospitalizations per person and family, respectively, with at least one hospitalization. Then, using the same calculation method we used for outpatient visits, we estimate that there would be an increase of 17 MTF admissions and a decrease of 5 CHAMPUS admissions per 1,000 beneficiaries in the expanded-MTF case. The tradeoff factor is 3.4—double the outpatient tradeoff factor.

In both cases, CHAMPUS utilization and costs vary more across program types (standard, CRI, CAM) than does MTF utilization. The catchment-area outpatient utilization rates shown in Table 23 for the baseline case, which are based on CRI, are 18 percent higher than the rates we measure in the standard program; if we were to simulate a CAM program instead, the baseline rates would be 7 to 10 percent higher than the standard program (not shown). In contrast, CHAMPUS inpatient utilization rates are lower in the managed-care programs; the baseline probabilities of hospitalization with CRI, as shown in Table 24, are 25 percent lower than without managed care. This pattern of higher outpatient utilization and lower inpatient utilization is characteristic of HMO plans.

CHAMPUS Costs

The 9 percent decrease in CHAMPUS costs that we predict for case 2 (versus case 1) is slightly lower than the percentage decrease in CHAMPUS utilization. Table 25 shows per-family costs and total program costs in the two cases—first costs to DoD and then total costs to all payers. The latter, which include payments by CHAMPUS and others for all costs allowed by CHAMPUS, exclude billed charges that exceed CHAMPUS fee limits and services not covered by CHAMPUS. These cost estimates have been adjusted for incompleteness and include administrative costs, as mentioned earlier in this section.

---

[10]Viewed from a government-wide perspective, there is presumably an offsetting decrease in Medicare-financed utilization by beneficiaries 65 and older.

Table 25

**CHAMPUS Cost in Baseline and Expanded Cases (1 & 2) (FY 1992
and 1997 MTFs and U.S. populations)**

Beneficiary Category	Government Paid		Total Cost	
	Baseline (1)	Expanded MTF (2)	Baseline (1)	Expanded MTF (2)
1992				
Cost/family	$1,428	$1,299	$1,739	$1,578
AD dependents	1,492	1,342	1,607	1,454
Retirees & deps.	1,363	1,255	1,871	1,739
Total cost (bil.)	$3.14	$2.86	$3.82	$3.47
1997				
Cost/family	$1,446	$1,318	$1,782	$1,619
AD dependents	1,480	1,315	1,592	1,421
Retirees & deps.	1,419	1,320	1,937	1,781
Total cost (bil.)	$3.20	$2.92	$3.95	$3.59

Like CHAMPUS utilization, costs for the baseline case vary with the managed-care program we simulate. There are few differences in the results for 1992 and 1997; cost per household is higher in 1997 because more beneficiaries live in noncatchment areas, but the total population is smaller and so total costs are almost the same. Total CHAMPUS costs paid by DoD for case 1 (with CRI) are predicted to be 11 percent higher than actual estimated costs for FY92, which were $2.83 billion for beneficiaries living in the United States. Two studies conclude that the benefits changes DoD has made in its new CRI programs and other changes expected to affect costs should largely eliminate these higher costs in the future (Congressional Budget Office, 1993; Lewin-VHI, 1993a and 1993b).

Although not shown here, we did use our regression results to simulate a CAM program instead of CRI, based on the limited CAM data we had. Using CAM as the model for managed care, we predict that CHAMPUS costs would be closer to actual costs for FY92. As suggested earlier, the CAM estimates may be influenced by other factors, since we have data for only one Navy site and one Air Force site. However, we can use the CAM results as an indication of what the CHAMPUS savings in case 2 would be in a less costly program than CRI. With CAM, we would still predict a drop in CHAMPUS costs of 8 percent in case 2—a savings of about $230 million instead of $282 million for the CRI case.

Total costs, including those paid by the beneficiary and other insurance as well as DoD, are over 20 percent higher than DoD costs alone. The difference is considerably smaller for active-duty dependents (8 percent) than for other beneficiaries (37 percent) because the CHAMPUS benefits for active-duty

66

personnel are more generous and because such beneficiaries are much less likely to have private insurance.[11] Compared with those in case 1, total allowed costs are $352 million, or 9 percent, lower in case 2 with CRI.

---

[11]For both groups, the difference between DoD costs and allowed costs would be higher without managed care.

6. Utilization and Costs in Cases with Commercial Health Plans

As Congress directed, some of the cases studied included commercial health plans, which would constitute the only health care source for enrollees. It is not possible to predict the costs of these plans from CHAMPUS data because, for most beneficiaries, CHAMPUS augments the MTFs and/or private health plans and is rarely the sole source of care. Instead, we predicted costs for the cases that included stand-alone civilian plans from civilian-sector data. Since beneficiaries would generally have a choice of plans in these cases, our first step was to predict the health-plan choices of military beneficiaries if these cases were adopted.

To predict plan choice, we developed a two-part model of family health-plan choices using data from the beneficiary survey regarding preferences for military versus civilian plans and data from a national survey regarding choices between civilian HMOs and FFS plans. We used this model to predict, for cases 3 and 4, the fraction and types of military families who would choose each of the types of health plan envisioned.

We then estimated per-capita costs in each of the cases' health plans, based on the characteristics of the plans and the families they would enroll. We employed different costing methods for the three major types of health plans: (1) for commercial FFS plans, we predicted per-capita costs from an expenditure simulation model that predicts health care expenditures and plan costs for families with different characteristics and FFS plans with different benefit packages, (2) for commercial HMO plans, we used the premiums charged by HMOs offered through the Federal Employees Health Benefits Plan in different geographic areas, and (3) for MTF plans, we predicted outpatient and inpatient workloads, using the models developed for cases 1 and 2, which were then costed by IDA. FFS and MTF plan predictions were based on the characteristics of the families predicted to choose these types of plans. HMO costs do not necessarily reflect true costs for the military population expected to enroll in HMOs because we lacked the data necessary for estimating population-specific costs and many HMOs do not set different premiums for different enrolled populations. We estimated MTF workload levels for three scenarios: (1) the MTFs operate as they do now, (2) the MTFs charge a modest fee for each clinic visit, and (3) the MTFs operate as a staff-model HMO.

68

Appendix E gives more detailed descriptions of the analyses we conducted for cases 3 and 4. In the remainder of this section, we will summarize our analysis of plan choice in cases 3 and 4, and then of civilian-plan costs and MTF workloads. The section concludes with an estimate of the employer contributions for military beneficiaries under health reform, based on the Clinton proposal.

Plan Choice

Case 3 would offer military families a choice of commercial FFS and HMO plans, depending on what plans are available in each geographic area or can be induced to serve areas with sizeable military populations. To analyze this case requires predicting how many families, and which families, would choose an FFS plan and how many would choose an HMO. Case 4 adds to these two commercial choices a largely MTF-based plan in areas served by an MTF. We modeled this three-way choice as a sequential decision. First, families choose whether to enroll in one of the civilian plans or the MTF plan. Families that choose the civilian system then select either an FFS plan or an HMO. Therefore, both cases require an analysis of the choice between civilian FFS and HMO plans and case 4 requires a preceding analysis of the choice between civilian and MTF plans.

Choice Between the Civilian and Military Health Care Systems

To measure relative preferences for health plans that rely on the civilian versus the military system, the beneficiary survey asked respondents to indicate their potential interest in replacing their current health coverage with each of two hypothetical health plans. The hypothetical plans were both HMOs, requiring beneficiaries to obtain their care at or through MTFs or civilian providers. In all other respects, the plans were identical: They added preventive examinations and routine eye care to the current CHAMPUS benefit package and the only cost sharing was a $5-per-visit charge for outpatient visits. In addition, the plans guaranteed access to care within 0–3 days, depending on the type of care. For each plan—civilian or MTF—survey respondents were asked whether they would choose the new plan instead of their current military health coverage if the new plan charged them a premium of $75 a month, $50 a month, or nothing. Each respondent thus made six hypothetical choices, each between current benefits and one of the two new plans at one of three premium levels; we obtained 89,281 responses about preferences for hypothetical plans. (We reproduce the survey questions at the end of Appendix E.)

We use probit regression to estimate the relationship between the probability of choosing an MTF-based HMO over the current coverage and the probability of choosing a civilian HMO over the current coverage. We use these relationships, along with expected utility theory and its assumption that preferences are transitive, to predict families' preferences between the civilian and military health care systems. (Our methods are explained in detail in Appendix E.) To illustrate, suppose the model predicts that a family with specified characteristics prefers a civilian HMO to current care and prefers current care to the MTF-HMO. Then we can infer that the family would prefer the civilian HMO to the MTF-HMO. Although our survey questions do not explicitly ask about civilian fee-for-service plans, we assume that a family that prefers the civilian HMO to the MTF-HMO would also prefer a civilian fee-for-service plan to the military plan, and that a preference for the MTF-HMO over the civilian HMO would extend to a preference for the military plan over other civilian alternatives. These assumptions then allow us to use our estimated regression to predict preferences between the civilian and military health systems. Although our predictions are based on responses to hypothethical questions, the marketing and economic literatures provide some evidence that stated preferences do predict actual behavior (see Manning and Marquis, 1989, for a summary of some of that literature). The explanatory variables in our regression include:

- military service, age, sex, and race of the military sponsor;

- whether the family has insurance in addition to its military coverage;

- length of residence in the area;

- family income;

- health status and expected health care use in the future;

- whether the family's usual source of care is civilian or military;

- characteristics of the MTF(s) in the area;

- whether the new option is a civilian or military plan;

- the premium cost to enroll;

- interactions between the type of new option and family characteristics to capture any differences in system preferences for different types of families.

We estimated separate models for active-duty families, families of retirees under age 65, and families of retirees 65 and older. Since each respondent reported his or her choice for six different optional plans, we had multiple observations on the dependent variable for each family. We corrected for the intrafamily correlation resulting from the multiple observations.

The regression results are shown in the appendix in Tables E.1–E.3, which report the effect of a change in each explanatory variable on the probability of choosing the military HMO or the civilian HMO in preference to current military coverage.

There are similar patterns of findings across the different subgroups. Price is an important factor in all groups; a $10 per month increase in the cost of joining a new plan reduces the probability of selecting it by about 6 to 7 percentage points.[1] Those who currently use the MTF for most of their care are more likely to report they would join a military HMO and less likely to be interested in the civilian HMO than those who usually obtain their health care from civilian providers. In all three groups, male sponsors and families with insurance in addition to their military benefit are more likely to prefer the new civilian plan to their current military coverage; nonwhites and older sponsors in all groups are more likely to prefer the military HMO than others. In all three subgroups, families who expect to have a large number of physician visits are less willing to switch from their current CHAMPUS or military plan into either of the new options. Perhaps those who expect to need care are reluctant to change providers and believe that a change in plan would entail such a provider change. Although not completely consistent across all subgroups, there is a tendency for persons who expect to have a hospitalization to be more likely to express a willingness to switch into one of the new plans; since the new plans required no cost sharing for inpatient care, this finding may reflect the effect of expected out-of-pocket payments on plan preferences.

We used the estimated model to simulate whether active-duty and retired families would choose a military plan or a civilian plan using methods described in Appendix E. Table 26 illustrates our results, assuming that all military personnel have the military HMO option available. In actual implementation of our model, our simulations restrict the choice of the military option to families in catchment areas (see the discussion below), and consequently the probabilities shown in Table 26 overstate predicted enrollment in the MTF-based plan under case 4. However, our intention here is to illustrate the findings and the role of personal characteristics on choices, without confounding the opportunity set with these characteristics. For the results in Table 26, we have replicated each family's choice 50 times. The proportion selecting the military option shown is the average proportion over the 50 replications.

---

[1]The change in probability is evaluated at the mean probability for the subgroup.

Table 26

**Percentage of Families Selecting Military Versus Civilian Plan
by Premium Level, Health Status, and Usual Source of Care**

	Dependents of Active-Duty Personnel	Retirees Under Age 65	Retirees Age 65 and Older
Premium level for civilian plan[a]			
$0	27	30	40
$20 single/$50 family	68	70	66
$30 single/$75 family	82	86	76
Health status of sickest family member			
Excellent	68	69	64
Good	69	70	66
Fair	68	73	67
Poor	62	77	66
Usual source of care			
Civilian	60	63	60
Military	70	80	74

[a]Cost of military plan assumed zero. Military and civilian options assumed available to all families.

The choice of system is responsive to differences in the premium cost to beneficiaries. The arc elasticity of demand implied by the choices shown in Table 26 for the two positive premiums for the civilian plan is –0.6. This means that a 1 percent increase in the premium level for the civilian plan leads to a 0.6 percent decrease in the probability of choosing that plan. This compares quite favorably to the price elasticity of demand estimates based on observed choices of nonmilitary personnel, which range from –0.16 to –0.54 (Marquis, Kanouse, and Brodsley, 1985; Manning and Marquis, 1989).

Selection effects—differences in plan choice by health status—differ among the subpopulations. There is some small, favorable health selection into the military plan by active-duty dependents, in contrast to adverse selection among the retirees under age 65. These differences are the total effects of health status and other characteristics that vary with health on choices. The net effects of health status controlling for other characteristics also show similar patterns (see the marginal effects from the probit regression parameters given in Appendix E). Not surprisingly, the preference for the military HMO is much higher among those for whom the military currently provides most of the care.

72

Choice Among Civilian Systems

For the second stage of our sequential decisionmaking model, we used data from the 1987 National Medical Expenditure Survey (NMES) to estimate a model of choice between civilian FFS and HMO plans. The NMES was a panel survey that was administered to a cross section of the civilian, noninstitutional population to measure health-insurance coverage, health status and health care use.

The sample for our estimation was limited to families with an insured, working family head who had a choice of health-insurance plans from his or her employer. The estimation sample included 1,508 families. We limited the sample in this way to model the FFS-HMO enrollment decision among families who had the opportunity to enroll in an HMO. Our criterion, however, imperfectly selects those families who have this opportunity. For some families who have a choice of insurance plans, the choice will be among high- and low-option FFS plans. For others, the choice may be between an FFS plan and some managed-care plan other than an HMO. However, the data available to us do not provide the information to make more accurate selections.

We used a probit regression, similar to the regression used for the military-civilian choice model, to estimate the relationship between family characteristics and the decision to enroll in an HMO instead of an FFS plan.[2] Our model results are given in Table E.4. Male, educated, and nonwhite primary insureds are more likely to elect an HMO. The coefficient estimates also suggest some adverse health selection into the HMO, but the health status effects are not statistically significant.

Simulating Health-Plan Choices for Cases 3 and 4

For case 3, we simulated the choice between a civilian FFS plan and a civilian HMO, using the model we estimated from the NMES data and simulation methods described in Appendix E. As we described above, the HMO enrollment rate we measured in the NMES probably underestimates enrollment in a population able to choose an HMO. In our estimation sample, 25 percent of families were enrolled in an HMO. Other data from the Bureau of Labor Statistics (BLS), however, suggest that actual HMO enrollments are about 35 percent when employees are offered this type of plan. Enrollment in CRI Prime and the Air Force's CAM program, which offer benefits similar to a civilian HMO's benefits, also exceeded 30 percent after several years. Therefore, we

---

[2]We do not have details about the benefits or costs of the options that the family faces to include in our estimation model.

adjusted our probit model to result in predicted probabilities of HMO enrollment that accord with the BLS overall estimate of 35 percent.[3]

To predict choices for case 4, we combined the two choice models we estimated to form a sequential decision model in which military families first choose whether to enroll in the MTF plan or one of the civilian plans and then, if they choose a civilian plan, between FFS and HMO. These choices are assumed to be available to all families residing in MTF catchment areas; in other areas, families may choose only between the two types of civilian plans. Our approach assumes that the choice of civilian plans is independent of whether an MTF plan is among the options available to the family. While this is a strong and untestable assumption, we believe it is reasonable to assume that families' first choice is whether they want to receive care from military or civilian providers and that relative preferences among civilian alternatives are similar for military personnel living in catchment areas and those not in catchment areas.

Table 27 presents our simulation results for active-duty dependents (we assumed all active-duty personnel are automatically enrolled in the MTF plan) and for families of retirees under age 65.[4] The simulations assume that, to enroll in a civilian health plan, beneficiaries pay a premium contribution (either $20 or $30 a month for single coverage and $50 or $75 a month for family coverage); those enrolling in the MTF plan pay nothing. At current utilization levels, a $20/$50 premium differential would be necessary to assure that enough beneficiaries enroll in the MTF plan to sustain the current MTF system.

Table 27

Military Families' Plan Choices for Case 4

	Civilian Plan			Military
	FFS	HMO	Medicare	Plan
Active-duty dependents				
$20 single/$50 family premium	28%	15%		57%
$30 single/$75 family premium	20%	11%		69%
Retirees, dependents under 65				
$20 single/$50 family premium	38%	17%		47%
$30 single/$75 family premium	31%	14%		55%
Retirees, dependents 65 and over				
$20 per person premium			60%	40%
$32 per person premium			52%	48%

Note: Those not in catchment areas assumed to choose between civilian plans only.

[3]Since our cost estimates for civilian FFS and HMO plans were similar, this adjustment had little effect on estimated costs for alternative 3.

[4]We did not simulate choice of the civilian HMO among older retirees but rather assumed that they would select HMOs at the selection rate of other Medicare beneficiaries.

Civilian Plan Costs for Cases 3 and 4

To estimate the costs for beneficiaries who enroll in a civilian fee-for-service plan, we used a health expenditures simulation model previously developed by RAND. This model predicts individual and family health-plan expenditures as a function of the structure of the fee-for-service insurance plan; both plan and out-of-pocket expenditures are estimated. As described further in Appendix E, the model is based on the results of the RAND Health Insurance Experiment. The experiment was conducted in the 1970s and 1980s to determine the effects of cost sharing on health care demand. For this study, we updated the experimental data to 1990 using the National Medical Expenditures Survey and then to 1992 using the medical component of the Consumer Price Index. We ran the simulation for three CHAMPUS beneficiary groups: all eligibles, those predicted to enroll in a civilian fee-for-service plan in case 3, and those predicted to enroll in case 4. We assumed that the benefits in this civilian plan would resemble the current CHAMPUS benefits shown in Table 1, but we also simulated costs for retirees for a benefit package similar to the Clinton Administration's proposed Health Security Act. We included a 5 percent administrative loading fee in all simulations.

For beneficiaries predicted to enroll in a civilian HMO plan, we used the premiums currently paid for HMOs in the Federal Employees Health Benefits Plan (FEHBP). We analyzed the data for all HMOs offered in 1991 to determine whether there were significant differences in premium costs by geographic region. Although the premiums do vary from plan to plan, there was little regional variation in the median premium. Therefore, we simply set the costs of HMO enrollees in cases 3 and 4 at the median of FEHBP premiums for 1992, including the government and employee contributions.

For Medicare eligibles, we also needed a rough estimate of Medicare costs for those not enrolling in an MTF plan. We used per-capita Medicare costs for 1992, calculated from data reported in the 1993 Statistical Supplement to the Social Security Bulletin (U.S. Department of Health and Human Services, 1993). We set total costs equal to average charges plus administrative costs and government costs as average reimbursements plus administrative costs.

Even though many more beneficiaries are predicted to enroll in a fee-for-service plan in case 3 (there is no MTF plan), the estimated cost per person is relatively unaffected (Table 28). In either case, dependents of junior enlisted personnel incur higher expenditures than other active-duty personnel because the

Table 28

Civilian Plan Costs for Projected Enrolled Populations in Cases 3 and 4
(1992)

Type of Plan	Members of Families by Sponsor Type				
	All <65	Jr. Enlisted	Other Active Duty	Retired (<65)	Retired (65+)
FFS—cost per person					
Case 3					
Paid by plan		$1,967	$1,736	$2,201	
Out-of-pocket covered		109	149	529	
Out-of pocket uncov'd.		118	62	134	
Case 3—Clinton					
Paid by plan				$2466	
Out-of-pocket covered				498	
Out-of-pocket uncov'd.				84	
Case 4					
Paid by plan		$1,835	$1,730	$2,175	
Out-of-pocket covered		106	146	529	
Out-of pocket uncov'd.		141	81	134	
HMO—avg. premium per covered household					
Single coverage	$1,850				
Family coverage	4,625				
Medicare					
Paid by plan					$3,075
Not paid by plan					2,820

Note: "Out-of-pocket covered" costs are the deductible and copayment costs for services covered by the plan. "Out-of-pocket uncovered" costs are for services not covered by the plan.

deductibles they face are lower and they include spouses of childbearing age and infants. Despite the higher copayment they must pay, expenditures for retired family members are high because they are older. That the Clinton health plan's benefits are better than current CHAMPUS retiree benefits can be seen from the higher plan expenditures for the Clinton plan. HMO costs are not much different from fee-for-service plan costs, at least if the FEHBP premiums reflect what DoD's premiums would be for civilian HMOs.

Utilization in the MTF Plan in Case 4

We adapted the methods we used for cases 1 and 2 to estimate utilization for beneficiaries predicted to enroll in the MTF plan in case 4. In this case, recall that beneficiaries can enroll in *either* a civilian plan or an MTF plan, but they may not obtain health care from both. The MTF would provide all the health care for its enrollees, either directly or by arranging for and financing care from civilian providers. Therefore, we based our prediction of MTF utilization in case 4 on the total health utilization—civilian plus military—observed in areas where MTF capacity is large relative to the population served. We also estimated how this utilization would be different if the MTF plan operated like a civilian HMO or required that the patient share in the costs of care.

The first step in our analysis for case 4 was to reestimate the utilization regressions for cases 1 and 2, substituting the total number of civilian and military visits and admissions reported by survey respondents. We used the survey data on civilian utilization, rather than CHAMPUS records, because we wanted to include civilian utilization not financed through CHAMPUS. The regressions are reported in Tables E.6 through E.8.

To simulate non-active-duty utilization in case 4's MTF plans, *assuming no change in MTF operations or benefits*, we used the same general prediction method we used for the expanded MTF case 2. We did not use case 2's expanded list of MTFs, but we assumed the same high levels of beds per capita and staff (FTEs) per bed and a managed-care approach similar to CRI. We held active-duty utilization constant at current levels.

We then conducted a sensitivity analysis to determine how the utilization levels of non-active-duty MTF enrollees might vary—for example, if the MTF were to operate like a civilian HMO or charge its enrollees fees for care. (We continued to hold active-duty utilization constant.) For the HMO case, we substituted the HMO visit and admission rates we estimated for military beneficiaries from the National Health Interview Survey in Section 3. We based our estimates on the decrease in the number of health care episodes, relative to the number of episodes with free care, in the Health Insurance Experiment (HIE) for three different levels of cost sharing: (1) 25 percent for all services, (2) 10 percent for outpatient visits (approximately equivalent to a $15 clinic fee, and (3) 5 percent for outpatient services. The HIE results showed that cost sharing reduced the number of episodes generated by patients, but had little effect on the cost per episode. Therefore, the percentage decrease in utilization with cost sharing is predicted by the percentage decrease in episodes (Keeler et al., 1988).

Table 29 shows the average number of visits and the probability of having any inpatient care in the MTF plan for beneficiaries predicted to enroll in that plan in case 4. Visit rates are lower for all beneficiary groups in the HMO and cost-sharing cases, although the HMO levels are only slightly lower for retirees and dependents under 65. The probability of hospitalization drops in the civilian HMO scenario, especially for active-duty dependents, and there are more modest decreases for the scenario that would charge patients the equivalent of a 25 percent cost share. Charging nuisance fees for outpatient visits does decrease the average number of visits, but not the probability of hospitalization. Given the

Table 29

Utilization for MTF Enrollees

	Active-Duty Dependents	Retirees & Dependents	
		Under 65	65 & Over
Average visits			
Current MTF levels	4.03	3.60	5.88
Civilian HMO levels	2.92	3.36	4.51
25% for all services	3.02	2.70	4.41
10% for visits	3.30	2.95	4.82
5% for visits	3.47	3.10	5.06
Probability of any inpatient care			
Current MTF levels	0.142	0.111	0.238
Civilian HMO levels	0.076	0.092	0.180
25% for all services	0.107	0.083	0.179
10% for visits	0.142	0.111	0.238
5% for visits	0.142	0.111	0.238

range of estimates in Table 29, we conclude that utilization levels in an exclusive MTF plan are uncertain; with incentives to control utilization, military beneficiaries might decrease their high utilization rates to those of their civilian counterparts.[5]

As we did for cases 1 and 2, we adjusted these utilization figures for the differences between the survey data and the workloads reported by the MTFs, multiplied them by the total eligible population, and sent estimates of MTF workloads to IDA for costing.

Employer Contributions Under the Clinton Health Proposal

The Clinton health reform proposal included an employer mandate that would require most employers to contribute 80 percent of the cost of health insurance for their employees. To explore the effects of an employer mandate on military health costs, we estimated the contributions that would be required for working military beneficiaries under the provisions of the proposed legislation. Of course, these are not the only provisions possible, but we did not attempt to estimate contributions for other provisions.

---

[5]The HIE did not find that decreases in utilization with cost sharing led to lower health status for most persons. See Appendix E for a brief summary of these results and Newhouse (1994) for a report on the experiment.

Under the Clinton Plan, an employer would have been required to pay an amount for each employee that depends on the type of family (single person, married couple, one-parent family, two-parent family) and the number of hours worked. Hours worked were translated into fraction of FTE using a formula specified in Title I, Subtitle J, Section 1902 of the Health Security Act: hours worked in a month/120. In its report on the plan, the Congressional Budget Office (1994) calculated the average employer share per FTE in 1994 dollars.[6] Title VIII, Subtitle A, of the proposed legislation authorized DoD to collect employer contributions for its beneficiaries who choose a DoD health plan (MTF-based or civilian) instead of obtaining care through a health alliance.

We estimated the employer contributions that would be paid for all military beneficiaries to be $5 billion. The calculation is a simple one—the number of FTE workers in each family type times the employer contribution per FTE for that family type.

We determined the number of military families of each of the four types defined in the legislation from the beneficiary survey (Table 30). For active-duty families, we did not include the sponsor in defining family type because we assumed that DoD and not the family's health plan would provide active-duty health care. Therefore, we assumed that employers would be able to pay single-parent rates for active-duty families with two parents.

We estimated the number of FTEs for each group from the beneficiary survey and Current Population Survey (CPS) data. The beneficiary survey provides

Table 30

Distribution of Military Families by Type

Family Type	Family's Sponsor		
	Jr. Enlisted	Other Active Duty	Retired <65
Single	24.3%	10.8%	4.4%
2 adults	—	—	46.1%
1 adult+children	65.6%	83.9%	1.3%
2 adults+children	—	—	48.2%
Children only	10.1%	5.3%	—

Note: We assumed that benefits for active-duty personnel would not be recovered from their spouses' civilian employers. Therefore, we treated active-duty families with two adults as having only one adult.

---

[6]We used CBO's figures because they were the only publicly available figures that actually derived employer contributions in addition to health-plan premiums. The two differ because of families with two workers.

hours worked by category (35+, 20–34, <20, variable) for sponsors (retired only) and spouses. Self-employed workers are a separate category, and so no hours were recorded for them. Those working 35+ hours are counted as full-time workers. To determine the number of FTEs for the part-time categories, we used the mean number of hours worked from the CPS within the range for the two part-time categories: 26.4 and 9.4 hours (these figures did not differ by sex).[7] Since working less than 120 hours a month is relatively uncommon, changing the values for part-time workers would not have much effect on these calculations. Our initial calculations did not include contributions for those reporting variable hours or who are self-employed, so our estimates are somewhat conservative— especially for retired families. When we counted all self-employed as full-time workers and included variable-hour workers in the lowest part-time group, our estimate of contributions increased to $5.5 billion.

_____

[7]We did not include that fraction of the workers in the <20-hours category estimated from the CPS to have worked fewer than 40 hours per month because the legislation does not define them as part-time employees.

7. Conclusions

All groups of military beneficiaries are heavier users of medical care than are comparable civilian populations. The research on the effects of cost sharing on health care demand suggests that much of the difference—30–40 percent for outpatient visits and 20–30 percent for the fraction hospitalized—can be attributed to the availability of free care in MTFs. However, other factors may also be playing a role: a higher incidence of certain health conditions (e.g., injuries) coupled with an emphasis on health maintenance for active-duty personnel, frequent family separations, and the incentive inherent in medical resource allocation to maximize MTF workload counts.

If free MTF care is an important factor, as seems likely, expanding the availability of MTF care should increase quantity demanded. Our analysis of the 1992 Military Beneficiary Survey data shows that CHAMPUS-eligible beneficiaries respond to higher MTF resource levels (beds and staff) by increasing their MTF utilization and decreasing their CHAMPUS utilization. However, the MTF increase is considerably larger than the CHAMPUS decrease—70 percent higher for outpatient care and 150 percent higher for inpatient care. Medicare-eligible beneficiaries also use more MTF services. We were not able to estimate the change in their civilian utilization, but any civilian-sector savings now accrue to Medicare rather than the MHSS.

This finding that demand for MHSS services increases with the availability of free care is supported by previous reports on DoD's experience with two programs that increased the availability of free or almost-free care: PRIMUS/NAVCARE clinics, in which civilian contractors provide primary care to military beneficiaries, and the CHAMPUS Reform Initiative, which offered an enrollment option with low CHAMPUS charges. Both programs led to increased utilization (Kennell et al., 1991, and Hosek et al., 1993).

How beneficial is the added health care used when MTF care is more readily available? Answering this difficult question was beyond the scope of this study. The health-insurance experiment conducted in the 1970s invested a considerable effort to assess the relationship between health care use and health status. After three to five years, individuals given more generous insurance used considerably more care, but there were at most small changes in their health status (Brook et al., 1984). Most of the improvements observed were for the poor.

The MTF system was built to support the medical requirements for wartime. With these requirements declining in the post–Cold War era, DoD could consider a major structuring of the MTF system, limiting its role in providing peacetime health care and offering commercial health plans instead to some or all non-active-duty beneficiaries. Our analysis of beneficiary preferences suggests that many might prefer civilian plans, *provided that there was no erosion of benefits in these plans.* A comparison of the costs in a restructured system and in the current system requires that our results be combined with the results of IDA's research; in preparing its report to Congress on the Comprehensive Study of the Military Health Care System (Department of Defense, 1994), PA&E did combine these results and concluded that DoD should size its MTF system to meet the peacetime demand from military beneficiaries only if it can control this demand through a combination of initiatives.

Appendix

A. Survey Weights

Overview of Method

We calculated survey weights to ensure that our utilization and cost estimates would reflect the characteristics of the population from which the sample was drawn, assuming simple random sampling within cells. Using the parametric approach to calculating nonresponse weights as described below allowed us to account for differential rates of response (e.g., by sponsor race) that were not included in the weights provided with the survey data.

Our approach to weighting proceeded in two steps. First, we calculated weights based on the sampling fraction from the survey design:

$$w_j = \text{(number in population in cell } j)/\text{(number sampled in cell } j)$$

where w_j is the inverse of the sampling fraction. Cells indexed by j are defined in the sampling grid by sponsor status and region. Second, we calculated nonresponse weights from a logistic regression with response status as the dependent variable and independent variables reported on the survey header.[1] The nonresponse weight, γ_i for household i is calculated as $1/\hat{p}_i$ where

$$1 - \hat{p}_i = \frac{e^{(\alpha + \Sigma \beta_\ell X_{i\ell})}}{1 + e^{(\alpha + \Sigma \beta_\ell X_{i\ell})}} \tag{1}$$

Here, $1 - \hat{p}_i$ is the probability of nonresponse, and $\hat{p}_i$ is the probability of response.

The weight for household i in cell j is the product of $w_{j_{(i)}} * \gamma_i$, scaled by a multiplicative constant, k, where

$$k = \# \ respondents \ / \ \sum_i (\gamma_i \times w_{j_{(i)}}) \ .$$

---

[1]Separate models were fit for active-duty sponsors and retirees/survivors since information was missing for all non-active-duty sponsors for some potential predictors of nonresponse: education, race, and number of dependents.

84

This scales the weights to the original sample size. Omitting k, the household weights would then sum to the total population of households.

Sampling Weights

Sampling weights, 1/sampling fraction, are reported in Table A.1. The reader is referred to Lurie et al. (1994) for details regarding survey sampling methods for this study.

Nonresponse Analyses

A total of 44,293 sponsors were included in the survey sample. Of these, 58.7 percent were respondents, 17.2 percent were postal return nonrespondents, and 24.1 percent were other nonrespondents or refusals. A 0/1 logit model was specified, categorizing respondents (0) versus all categories of nonresponse (1). Model coefficients are reported in Tables A.2 (active duty) and Table A.3 (retirees, survivors).

For each predictor variable, the odds ratio for nonresponse versus response, controlling for other predictor variables in the model, is given by the antilog (the exponential) for the estimated logit regression coefficient. For a dichotomous predictor variable such as "FEMALE," this leads to the odds ratio for the two groups defined by the predictor variable (FEMALES versus MALES). For a continuous predictor variable such as AGE, this leads to the odds ratio for two groups that differ by one unit on the predictor variable.

Active-Duty Households

Overall, 51 percent of active-duty households were respondents and 49 percent were included in one of the nonresponse categories.

Positive relationships between sponsor characteristics and probability of nonresponse were identified for the following variables: reservists, blacks, and those sampled from the Tricare-Tidewater and Air Force CAM regions.

Negative relationships between sponsor characteristics and probability of nonresponse were found for the following: age, female, married, those sampled from Army CAM locations, and all other service-rank groups.

These rates control for other predictors in the model. The joint effects of these variables can be calculated using equation 1. For illustration, the estimated probability of nonresponse for an unmarried, nonblack male, age 20, Navy

Table A.1

Sampling Weights

Region	Beneficiary Group					
	E1–E4 w/Deps.	E5–E9 w/Deps.	Officer w/Deps.	E1–E4 No Deps.	E5–E9 No Deps.	Officer No Deps.
Army CAM	1832.9	6945.6	3723.8	3051.8	732.4	1061.9
CRI	11834.0	42333.6	15429.5	19867.6	9288.5	5336.2
Army GTC	7963.1	27402.9	9572.0	12971.3	3775.3	3287.7
Tricare	2631.7	11662.0	4597.9	2957.0	2305.6	662.0
Overlapping	8113.9	34695.0	21833.1	9217.2	6687.8	5638.6
Southeast PPO	5336.4	22175.8	8988.3	5139.4	4356.1	2604.2
New Orleans CRI	73.0	534.8	175.0	—	101.5	86.0
PRIMUS/NAVCARE	6947.8	19414.3	7267.8	7384.8	3321.5	2520.1
Noncatchment	2832.0	12601.3	4477.4	2968.2	2084.4	1145.6
Overseas	17162.5	58800.4	17056.2	17712.4	9845.9	5477.2
Navy CAM	782.7	2913.9	740.8	931.3	369.2	153.6
Air Force CAM	735.4	1910.1	631.5	291.0	416.3	184.0
No initiatives	17339.1	45190.6	17055.4	18439.8	8199.8	4806.3
Naval afloat	10926.7	39672.3	9018.6	23410.6	12037.9	4364.2

Table A.1—continued

Region	Beneficiary Group					
	Retirees Under 65	Retirees Over 65	Reserve Ret. <65	Reserve Ret. 65+	Survivor Under 65	Survivor Over 65
Army CAM	13134.7	4296.0	145.6	435.6	—	536.8
CRI	89638.7	52174.1	3540.6	13660.4	2417.7	13709.1
Army GTC	43374.2	14005.6	1356.8	3569.7	2468.7	2521.2
Tricare	21824.1	6815.9	236.7	794.3	1335.0	1348.3
Overlapping	95135.1	43563.7	6110.3	15622.7	4269.7	8289.6
Southeast PPO	106830.5	47111.0	5467.9	14173.0	2682.7	8679.3
New Orleans CRI	2275.0	865.1	237.3	538.0	—	—
PRIMUS/NAVCARE	52716.6	20249.7	1599.2	5124.5	1618.5	4313.2
Noncatchment	183127.0	66836.8	17569.0	37394.0	6777.2	14114.6
Overseas	10922.2	2800.0	626.4	758.1	—	233.0
Navy CAM	6032.5	1677.2	133.3	325.0	337.0	301.5
Air Force CAM	14642.7	6206.9	610.3	1899.2	648.0	981.0
No initiatives	102706.1	34110.9	6307.1	13303.8	1964.9	5866.3
Naval afloat	—	—	—	—	—	—

Table A.2

**Logistic Regression of Nonresponse for
Active-Duty Sponsors**

Variable	Parameter Estimate	Standard Error
Intercept	1.7747	0.0755
Air Force Reserve	0.1180	0.0837
Army Reserve	0.1231	0.0830
Navy Reserve	0.3015	0.0833
Age	–0.0327	0.0024
Female	–0.3512	0.0450
Black	0.5018	0.0349
Married	–0.0729	0.0361
Army CAM	–0.1565	0.0532
Tricare	0.2853	0.0519
Air Force CAM	0.2615	0.0536
Army E5–E9	–0.6886	0.0610
Army officer	–0.5915	0.0753
Navy E1–E4	–0.2843	0.0592
Navy E5–E9	–0.9817	0.0585
Navy officer	–1.3617	0.0675
Air Force E1–E4	–0.9804	0.0590
Air Force E5–E9	–1.2919	0.0657
Air Force officer	–1.1589	0.0713

Table A.3

**Logistic Regression of Nonresponse for
Retirees/Survivors**

Variable	Parameter Estimate	Standard Error
Intercept	6.4820	0.4155
Navy	0.1052	0.0426
Air Force	–0.1137	0.0438
Age	–0.2636	0.0138
Age squared	0.0021	0.0001
Enlisted paygrade	0.5967	0.0413
Permanent disability	0.5403	0.0569
Temporary disability	–0.9361	0.2543
Survivor	1.3297	0.0881
Overseas	0.3294	0.0660

E1–E4 was 70 percent, while the estimated probability of nonresponse for a married, nonblack Air Force officer, age 30, was 39 percent.

Retirees, Survivors

For retirees and survivors, 74 percent were respondents and 26 percent were included in one of the nonresponse categories.

As indicated above, retirees generally showed lower rates of nonresponse than the active-duty sponsors. For example, the estimated probability of nonresponse for a retired, nondisabled Naval officer aged 50 residing in CONUS was 21 percent.

Postal Return Nonresponse

A separate set of household weights were calculated by IDA that excluded postal return nonrespondents from nonresponse weight calculations. This approach assumes that postal return nonrespondents are effectively missing "at random." To test this assumption an analysis of postal return nonresponse was performed.

Results suggest that predictors of postal returns show similar patterns to those for overall nonresponse for retirees/survivors. For active-duty sponsors, the effects of some demographic and location variables are similar between the models predicting postal returns and overall nonresponse. Other results are detailed below.

Differences between the two types of nonresponse for active-duty sponsors are shown in stronger effects for "region" and reversed directions of coefficients for Army E5–E9, Army officers, and Navy E1–E4 (Table A.4). Those with postgraduate education are less likely to be postal return nonrespondents, when no effect of educational level was found in the nonresponse model. Marital status was not a significant predictor of postal returns; however, other demographic variables (age, female, black) showed similar patterns to the combined nonresponse analysis. Data show that those sampled from Air Force CAM sites were more likely to be postal return nonrespondents. Controlling for this effect, Air Force officers were not significantly different from Army E1–E4 in likelihood of postal nonresponse.

For retirees/survivors, those in Air Force CAM sites were also more likely to be postal return nonrespondents. Otherwise, these predictors showed similar

Table A.4

**Logistic Regression of Postal Return Nonresponse
for Active-Duty Sponsors**

Variable	Parameter Estimate	Standard Error
Intercept	−0.6107	0.0824
Age	−0.0156	0.0027
Female	−0.1323	0.0512
Black	0.1389	0.0383
Graduate education	−0.1829	0.0570
Army CAM	−0.3576	0.0655
CRI	−0.2853	0.0629
Army Gateway to Care	−0.2074	0.0595
Tricare	0.3555	0.0624
Southeast PPO	0.2244	0.0598
New Orleans CRI	−0.6006	0.0959
PRIMUS/NAVCARE	−0.1730	0.0628
Noncatchment areas	0.2457	0.0604
Navy CAM	−0.1049	0.0699
Air Force CAM	0.2984	0.0651
Navy afloat	−0.5502	0.0730
Army E5–E9	0.1839	0.0573
Army officer	0.7006	0.0601
Navy E1–E4	0.2201	0.0638
Navy E5–E9	−0.3681	0.0643
Navy officer	−0.2922	0.0730
Air Force E1–E4	−0.4542	0.0599
Air Force E5–E9	−0.3759	0.0663
Air Force officer	0.0086	0.0648

relationships to postal return nonresponse as in the original nonresponse analyses (Table A.5).

Although some differences in models were noted, there does not appear to be compelling evidence to distinguish postal return nonrespondents from other nonresponse subjects in the survey design. Also, the assumption that postal returns are missing at random does not appear to be supported by the analyses reported here.

Tables A.6 and A.7 report the household weights we received with the data and the weights we calculated.

Table A.5

**Logistic Regression of Postal Return Nonresponse
for Retirees/Survivors**

Variable	Parameter Estimate	Standard Error
Intercept	2.4149	0.5711
Navy	0.3977	0.0159
Air Force	−0.0159	0.0765
Age	−0.1791	0.0195
Age squared	0.0014	0.0002
Enlisted paygrade	0.5859	0.0768
Permanent disability	0.6967	0.0852
Temporary disability	−0.1885	0.3020
Survivor	0.3179	0.1676
Overseas	0.6159	0.0990
Air Force CAM	0.3477	0.1129

Table A.6

Original Household Weights

	Beneficiary Group					
Region	E1–E4 w/Deps.	E5–E9 w/Deps.	Officer w/Deps.	E1–E4 No Deps.	E5–E9 No Deps.	Officer No Deps.
Army CAM	6384.9	12347.1	5408.1	9606.3	1874.2	1757.3
CRI	37894.5	70967.1	22965.2	64041.9	15055.2	9180.4
Army GTC	26488.0	54678.6	18503.7	45680.4	8991.6	5762.0
Tricare	8764.0	24549.0	7833.3	12317.8	5214.2	1932.5
Overlapping	21809.4	57893.8	34826.9	32113.6	12114.4	9999.0
Southeast PPO	13654.3	33915.3	15027.1	18738.4	5973.0	5167.1
New Orleans CRI	177.3	1008.0	258.1	—	181.1	87.5
PRIMUS/NAVCARE	20547.8	35657.1	11682.9	30791.3	5902.6	3584.2
Noncatchment	6867.8	20644.8	7113.2	8078.6	3452.6	1985.8
Overseas	51016.6	106954.0	27000.0	87873.6	22449.1	10241.3
Navy CAM	1823.7	4798.5	1052.9	2235.1	919.5	371.6
Air Force CAM	1555.2	3282.7	1123.7	1496.7	557.3	439.4
No initiatives	35663.9	71792.6	29111.4	44821.9	11304.1	9001.7
Naval afloat	35050.9	72626.8	13200.4	88108.9	21112.2	6611.3

Table A.6—continued

Region	Retirees Under 65	Retirees Over 65	Beneficiary Group Reserve Ret. <65	Reserve Ret. 65+	Survivor Under 65	Survivor Over 65
Army CAM	17828.3	5474.6	197.8	501.8	—	1362.3
CRI	139949.4	70440.2	3936.6	13781.3	5501.9	26826.3
Army GTC	64920.3	18448.4	1811.5	4627.9	4188.3	4954.6
Tricare	30479.4	9356.4	405.8	1021.5	696.8	3420.5
Overlapping	139143.6	60855.8	8753.1	14570.1	10941.1	21940.3
Southeast PPO	159011.3	63703.1	6728.3	14302.1	5008.2	18435.1
New Orleans CRI	3521.0	1319.5	304.3	710.2	—	—
PRIMUS/NAVCARE	76236.8	26656.2	1774.2	8185.5	3647.8	6801.5
Noncatchment	265920.6	94823.1	18333.3	43034.0	14317.7	29202.2
Overseas	17325.2	4472.3	728.3	1255.7		744.0
Navy CAM	8979.5	2217.3	95.2	414.2	637.6	679.7
Air Force CAM	20412.9	8267.1	608.6	2247.4	2122.1	2113.6
No initiatives	149279.7	47413.6	8470.4	12759.3	4643.6	15147.6
Naval afloat	—	—	—	—	—	—

Table A.7

RAND Household Weights

Region	Beneficiary Group					
	E1–E4 w/Deps.	E5–E9 w/Deps.	Officer w/Deps.	E1–E4 No Deps.	E5–E9 No Deps.	Officer No Deps.
Army CAM	5424.7	12567.5	6152.1	11910.7	1645.1	1914.5
CRI	33488.6	75754.3	24548.1	66245.9	17232.6	9190.2
Army GTC	29071.8	56711.3	19209.8	50720.1	8144.0	7553.4
Tricare	9546.3	23717.3	7738.9	12559.4	4965.7	1127.2
Overlapping	22782.3	62188.8	34796.6	31632.5	12498.4	9987.4
Southeast PPO	12550.3	37350.3	14598.0	16223.2	8474.1	4348.2
New Orleans CRI	232.0	982.8	254.6	—	282.0	139.8
PRIMUS/NAVCARE	20246.8	34955.1	11822.9	27297.7	6515.1	4668.0
Noncatchment	6758.8	22056.4	7345.7	7579.3	3605.5	2053.7
Overseas	47926.7	107795.3	30142.1	53006.3	18491.6	11484.3
Navy CAM	1855.0	4921.7	1122.3	2125.0	629.4	248.4
Air Force CAM	1615.5	3265.8	1081.5	607.3	746.2	394.6
No initiatives	36885.7	75148.5	28388.0	53246.3	13689.2	8206.5
Naval afloat	33864.5	70644.7	13596.8	78249.5	23055.4	7350.4

94

Table A.7—continued

Region	Retirees Under 65	Retirees Over 65	Beneficiary Group Reserve Ret. <65	Reserve Ret. 65+	Survivor Under 65	Survivor Over 65
Army CAM	18603.0	5653.5	178.5	551.9	—	1320.9
CRI	128511.6	71300.4	4333.4	17574.7	4976.5	29249.6
Army GTC	61747.2	19059.4	1712.7	4532.1	4864.2	5740.7
Tricare	31826.1	9184.2	292.9	1023.2	3217.7	3042.6
Overlapping	139318.8	58985.8	7691.6	19896.9	9138.5	18787.5
Southeast PPO	151492.0	62933.6	6851.6	18116.9	5776.0	18039.9
New Orleans CRI	3370.5	1172.7	294.3	685.0	—	—
PRIMUS/NAVCARE	76045.3	27252.1	1978.0	6500.8	5709.3	9018.4
Noncatchment	284415.5	90427.4	21872.7	47418.9	16947.0	30860.2
Overseas	17617.8	4308.7	836.7	1102.3	—	2665.5
Navy CAM	8602.2	2274.5	160.4	426.3	695.7	512.6
Air Force CAM	20326.9	8075.0	757.0	2447.1	1539.6	2102.6
No initiatives	144102.2	44940.5	7819.7	16938.6	4109.3	13225.7
Naval afloat	—	—	—	—	—	—

B. Military/Civilian Utilization Comparisons: Data and Methods

Data Sources

Military Beneficiary Survey

For the purposes of this study, a beneficiary survey was fielded to active-duty, retiree, and survivor households.[1] For one randomly selected family member, the survey asked for counts of visits and inpatient nights by location of care. These locations include: MTF, including clinic, hospital, or field/fleet hospital; PRIMUS or NAVCARE clinic; civilian providers; Veterans Administration hospitals; or other, unspecified locations. For active-duty sponsors, visits to military facilities for sick call are distinguished from visits for other medical reasons. For each source, respondents could indicate the number of visits up to "10 or more" during the previous year. Therefore, the survey underestimates the number of visits made by high-frequency users.

In addition to health-services measures, the beneficiary survey provides information regarding household socioeconomic status (household income, sponsor education) and health status for the randomly selected individual (5-point health status scale and number of acute and chronic health conditions).

National Health Interview Survey

Data for civilian utilization rates are taken from the National Health Interview Survey (NHIS). Fielded annually by the U.S. Public Health Service, this survey assesses health status and health-services utilization for a civilian noninstitutionalized sample of approximately 50,000 households and 120,000 individuals. The survey obtains the same information as the military survey on household socioeconomic status and health status for each individual in the household.

We selected the subsample of households from the NHIS that were covered by private insurance for comparisons to the military beneficiary survey. This

---

[1]While included in the survey, data for reservists and OCONUS beneficiaries are not included in this report.

required us to use the 1989 NHIS, as only this year's data collection contains information regarding insurance coverage. Since we found no secular trends in civilian outpatient use or inpatient admissions between 1987 and 1991, the 1987 data can be compared with the military survey. We randomly selected one person from each civilian household for this analysis. Thus, corrections for intracluster correlation in utilization within households are not required to adjust standard errors of estimates.

Methods

We estimated logistic regressions for the probability of any outpatient visits (Table B.1) and the probability of any inpatient admissions (Table B.4). Our exploratory analysis indicated that the military and civilian samples could be pooled. However, we could not pool the samples for the least-squares regressions we estimated to model the number of outpatient visits, conditional on any visits occurring. Therefore, we estimated separate models for the conditional number of visits for the military group (Table B.2) and the civilian group (Table B.3). The dependent variable for these regressions was the natural logarithm of number of visits.

Since the military survey permitted answers only up to 10 visits for each source of care, we truncated the data in both data sets to make them more comparable. We carried out the analysis with truncations at 10 and 30 visits. The results were similar, and so we report only the results for the truncation at 10.

We used the regression models to calculate the military and civilian utilization rates shown in Section 3 in Tables 2 and 3. The method we used in these calculations differed slightly for the outpatient and inpatient estimates. To estimate per-capita visits, we first predicted the probability that each person in the military sample would have any visits from the logistic regression model in Table B.1 if that person were:

- a military beneficiary,
- a civilian in an FFS plan, and
- a civilian in an HMO plan.

The next step was to estimate from the regression models in Table B.2 and B.3 the number of visits (s)he would have, conditional on having some visits, under the same three scenarios. For that person, we calculated the predicted number of visits in each scenario by multiplying the predicted probability of having any visits by the expected numbers of visits, conditional on having any. The final step was to calculate the average predicted number of visits within each military population group in each scenario.

To estimate the fraction with inpatient care in each of the three scenarios, we first predicted the probability of having any inpatient use for each individual in the military sample under that scenario. We then calculated the average probability of inpatient use within each military population group.

Regression Variables

Three measures were used in assessing health-services utilization: a 0/1 indicator of any outpatient care; a 0/1 indicator of any inpatient care; and number of outpatient visits winsorized[2] at 10.

Preliminary analyses showed that the relationship between utilization and age is nonlinear, and that it differs by gender. While other functional forms were considered to control for these demographic variables (e.g., modeling via splines, with separate terms by gender), the final models specify age by groups—ages 0–17, 18–44, and 45–64—with separate coefficients for males and females for each group. Separate models were fit for Medicare eligibles (beneficiaries over age 64).

Measures of health status include a five-point scale (excellent, very good, good, fair, poor) of self-reported health status and self-reported acute and chronic conditions.

Household income, educational attainment for head of household (civilian) or sponsor (military), and number in household are indicators of household socioeconomic status. Preliminary analyses showed that a linear specification was adequate for these variables.

For civilians, an indicator variable is included that distinguishes those covered by HMO plans from these covered by FFS plans. This indicator is present only for the non-Medicare population.

Finally, we included indicator variables for observations with missing socioeconomic or health status variables (Table B.5).

---

[2]Winsorization accumulates observations at a truncation point. See, for example, Amemiya, 1985.

Table B.1

Any Outpatient Visits, Military and Civilian Populations

Variable	Estimated Coefficient	Standard Error
Intercept	0.4686	0.1384
Civilian	−1.0321	0.0831
Ages 0–17	0.7833	0.0524
Ages 45–64	0.0916	0.0444
Female	0.4676	0.0393
Female, childbearing age	0.5056	0.0588
Active-duty indicator	0.6865	0.0687
Female active-duty indicator	−0.0802	0.2146
Junior enlisted	−0.4760	0.1478
Black	−0.3326	0.0902
Other ethnicity	−0.1736	0.1133
Black civilian	0.3041	0.1072
Other civilian	−0.2051	0.1436
Catchment	0.0592	0.0673
Health status (1=excellent, 5=poor)	0.2221	0.0188
Acute conditions	0.1891	0.0243
Chronic conditions	0.3400	0.0257
Military acute conditions	1.1094	0.0570
Military chronic conditions	0.0085	0.0693
Income	0.0056	0.0011
Education	0.0626	0.0066
Number in household	−0.0157	0.0130
HMO	0.1627	0.0422
Military missing condition	0.2182	0.0835
Civilian missing income	−0.0851	0.0552
Civilian missing education	−0.3337	0.1641
Military missing income	−0.1665	0.1743
Military missing education	−0.1585	0.1824
Civilian missing health status	−1.1878	0.2674
Civilian missing health status	−1.1878	0.2674
Number of Observations	33473	

Table B.2

**Log (Number of Outpatient Visits) Military Beneficiaries
with Some Visits Truncated at 10**

Variable	Estimated Coefficient	t-statistic
Intercept	0.7972	23.54
Ages 0–17	0.0761	5.26
Ages 45–64	–0.0089	–0.63
Female	0.0896	9.20
Female, childbearing age	0.0734	4.62
Active-duty indicator	–0.0245	–1.50
Female active-duty indicator	0.1792	5.81
Junior enlisted	–0.0272	–1.21
Black	0.0216	1.64
Other ethnicity	–0.0554	–2.98
Catchment	0.0324	3.55
Health status (1=excellent, 5=poor)	0.1474	34.63
Acute conditions	0.1277	27.77
Chronic conditions	0.1107	24.58
Income	0.0007	2.45
Education	0.0017	0.78
Number in household	–0.0252	–7.85
Military missing conditions	0.0229	2.71
Military missing income	0.0257	0.89
Military missing education	0.1333	5.55
Military missing health status	0.0361	0.97
Number of observations	12550	
R^2	0.1978	

100

Table B.3

**Log (Number of Outpatient Visits) Civilians with
Some Visits Truncated at 10**

Variable	Estimated Coefficient	t-statistic
Intercept	0.2908	10.63
Ages 0–17	0.1006	9.06
Ages 45–64	−0.0144	−1.20
Female	0.0853	9.17
Female, childbearing age	0.1866	14.11
Black	−0.1808	−14.23
Other ethnicity	−0.1169	−5.87
Health status (1=excellent, 5=poor)	0.2082	45.48
Acute conditions	0.0650	16.97
Chronic conditions	0.1303	29.83
Income	0.0014	5.27
Education	0.0093	5.91
Number in household	0.0195	−6.39
HMO (civilian only)	0.0272	3.16
Civilian missing income	−0.0591	−4.67
Civilian missing education	−0.0183	−0.38
Civilian missing health status	−0.1087	−1.59
Number of observations	14150	
R^2	0.1253	

Table B.4

Any Hospital Stays, Military and Civilian Populations

Variable	Estimated Coefficient	Standard Error
Intercept	−3.2653	0.1721
Civilian	−0.2494	0.0805
Ages 0–17	−0.3579	0.0808
Ages 45–64	0.1836	0.0673
Female	−0.0953	0.0536
Female, childbearing age	0.8251	0.0738
Active-duty indicator	−0.2056	0.0941
Female active-duty indicator	0.5406	0.1525
Junior enlisted	0.6701	0.1715
Black	0.0579	0.1022
Other ethnicity	−0.0749	0.1296
Black civilian	−0.2974	0.1405
Other civilian	0.0454	0.2016
Catchment	−0.0785	0.0666
Health status (1=excellent, 5=poor)	0.4209	0.0211
Acute conditions	0.0781	0.0263
Chronic conditions	0.2077	0.0232
Military acute conditions	0.1011	0.0403
Military chronic conditions	−0.0741	0.0346
Income	−0.0044	0.0015
Education	−0.0179	0.0093
Number in household	0.0887	0.0175
HMO (civilian only)	−0.1390	0.0701
Military missing conditions	0.5123	0.0570
Civilian missing income	−0.0294	0.0929
Civilian missing education	0.0894	0.2946
Military missing income	−0.2719	0.1931
Military missing education	0.2143	0.1661
Civilian missing health status	0.2959	0.5227
Military missing health status	0.2665	0.2126
Number of observations	33473	

Table B.5

Means and Standard Deviations for Regression Variables

Variable	Mean	Standard Deviation
Civilian indicator	0.540	0.498
Indicator age 0–17	0.212	0.409
Indicator age 45–64	0.291	0.454
Female indicator	0.501	0.500
Female childbearing age	0.198	0.399
Active-duty indicator	0.129	0.335
Female active-duty indicator	0.014	0.118
Junior enlisted	0.011	0.104
Black	0.103	0.304
Other ethnicity nonwhite	0.047	0.212
Black civilian	0.064	0.246
Civilian of other ethnicity	0.022	0.148
In catchment area	0.367	0.482
HMO	0.156	0.363
Income (in $1,000)	36.402	16.412
Education (in years)	13.804	2.620
Number in household	2.806	1.410
Health status (1=excellent, 5=poor)	1.953	0.985
Acute conditions scale	0.006	0.999
Chronic conditions scale	0.008	1.005
Acute conditions—military	0.006	0.678
Chronic conditions—military	0.006	0.682
Military missing conditions	0.146	0.353
Civilian missing income	0.067	0.250
Civilian missing education	0.006	0.079
Military missing income	0.010	0.100
Military missing education	0.010	0.098
Civilian missing health status	0.002	0.043
Military missing health status	0.007	0.082
Any outpatient visits	0.827	0.378
Any inpatient stays	0.084	0.277
Number of visits (range 0–10)	3.116	3.079

C. Regression Methods for Predicting Demand in Alternative Systems

In the subsequent discussion, we will use the following variables:

y_i = health expenditures (or utilization) for individual i,

x_i = vector of individual characteristics,

d_i = vector of military and civilian health care variables.

The goal of this analysis is to evaluate the impact of system changes (included in the vector d_i) on the mean level of health care expenditures (y_i) and to perform some simple policy simulations. To accomplish this task, we need to account for the nonnormal statistical properties of health data. In particular, the observed distribution of health care expenditures has a mass point at zero, and for positive values it has excess weight in the tail that is inconsistent with a truncated normal distribution. Because these data are similar to those found in the RAND Health Insurance Experiment, we employ similar methods (Manning et al., 1987; and Duan et al., 1982).

The following specification determines whether an individual has positive expenditures, where the subscript i has been suppressed for convenience:

$$I^* = x\alpha_x + d\alpha_d + \epsilon_I$$

$$\epsilon_I \sim N\,(0,1)$$

$$\text{If } \begin{pmatrix} I^* > 0 \\ I^* \leq 0 \end{pmatrix}, \text{ then we observe } \begin{pmatrix} y > 0 \\ y = 0 \end{pmatrix}.$$

Conditional on an observation of positive expenditures (or equivalently a realization of ϵ_I), we model the distribution of (log) expenditures as follows:

$$\log(y) \mid (y > 0) = xb_x + db_d + \epsilon_2$$

$$\epsilon_2 \mid y > 0 \sim F\left(0, \sigma^2\right)$$

where $F\left(0, \sigma^2\right)$ denotes a distribution (possibly nonnormal) with mean 0 and variance σ^2.

104

In this model, we assume x and d are nonstochastic.[1] The assumption of normality yields a convenient representation for the conditional mean of the untransformed expenditures:

$$E[y \mid z, y > 0] = \exp(z\beta)\gamma$$

$$\beta = (\beta_x, \beta_d); \quad z = (x, d); \quad \gamma = E[exp(\epsilon^2)],$$

where γ is the retransformation factor that adjusts the bias in taking the antilog for the logarithmic-scale prediction $z\beta$.

Therefore, the unconditional mean of y can be computed as

$$E[y \mid z] = \Phi(z\alpha)\exp(z\beta)\gamma$$

$$\alpha = (\alpha_x, \alpha_d),$$

where $\Phi(\bullet)$ denotes the standard normal cumulative distribution function.

Point Estimation

We estimate the two-part model sequentially. In the first stage, we use maximum likelihood techniques under the assumption of normality (weighted probit) to compute an estimate of α. In the second stage, we estimate ordinary least squares regressions with (log) utilization or cost level *for those individuals with positive use* as the dependent variable and the same covariates to get an estimate of β. We compute a consistent estimate for the retransformation factor, γ, using the smearing estimator.[2] As a result, we obtain a consistent estimate of the mean health care utilization or cost of an individual with demographic characteristics x_i and dummy specification d_i using

$$\hat{E}(y_i \mid z_i) = \hat{\mathrm{Prob}}(y_i > 0 \mid z_i)\hat{E}(y_i \mid z_i, y_i > 0) = \Phi\left(z_i'\hat{\alpha}\right)\exp\left(z_i'\hat{\beta}\right)\hat{\gamma}.$$

For policy simulation, we use the estimated coefficients to predict utilization and costs for the survey sample, weighted to reflect the total population. We first specify new values for the variables in the d vector of health-system variables, incorporating the changes we want to simulate. If $z_i \equiv (x_i, d_i)$, then $\hat{E}(y_i \mid z_i)$ denotes the mean level of expenditures for a particular survey participant. We

---

[1]The vector d contains dummy variables indicating membership in the CRI and CAM enrollment programs. Enrollment is endogenous to utilization because beneficiaries base their enrollment decision on expected utilization. We could not control for this endogeneity.

[2]The smearing estimator is the sample average of the exponentiated residuals (i.e., $\hat{\gamma} = \frac{1}{N} \Sigma \exp(\hat{\epsilon}_i)$). Duan (1983) discusses this estimator in detail.

can then construct the vector $z_i^* \equiv (x_i, d_i^*)$, where d_i^* differs from d_i only in that it incorporates the changes to be simulated. Thus, for example, z_i^* may be thought of as a pseudo-individual who differs from the original z_i only in that z_i^* is now in a CRI plan instead of the standard program or is now served by a new military hospital instead of no MTF. The quantity $\hat{E}(y_i|z_i^*)$ denotes the predicted utilization of this pseudo-individual under standard CHAMPUS. The difference $\hat{E}(y_i|z_i) - \hat{E}(y_i|z_i^*)$ represents the expected change in mean health care utilization for individual z_i under a changed system, relative to the baseline situation. If w_i denotes the population weight associated with a survey participant, then an overall estimate of the mean impact of the simulated change may be computed as

$$\Delta \equiv \frac{1}{\sum w_i} \sum_{i=1}^{k} w_i \left[\hat{E}(y_i|z_i) - \hat{E}(y_i|z_i^*) \right].$$

Tables C.1 to C.10 contain the point estimates and t-statistics for all equations estimated. Tables C.11 and C.12 contain weighted means and standard deviations.

Table C.1

MTF Use for CHAMPUS-Eligible Adults in Catchment Areas

Variable	Probability of Visits>0		No. Visits if Visits>0		Probability: Hosp. Nights>	
	Coefficient	Stand. Error	Coefficient	Stand. Error	Coefficient	Stand. Error
Intercept	-0.50330	0.22927	0.38089	0.15636	-1.42981	0.36598
Retired	-0.29566	0.11116	-0.29662	0.07706	-0.20371	0.17320
Retired female	0.09681	0.04334	0.10105	0.03254	-0.23984	0.07756
Officer	0.04218	0.05187	-0.00302	0.03651	—	—
Not MTF service	-0.23934	0.04119	0.03739	0.03041	-0.15897	0.07172
Employed	-0.11023	0.03959	-0.05859	0.02783	-0.21963	0.06382
Family income	0.00827	0.01746	-0.04684	0.01116	-0.02309	0.02295
Family size	0.07709	0.01462	0.03365	0.00946	0.01620	0.02229
Age	0.03372	0.00970	0.01183	0.00681	-0.01183	0.01592
Age squared	-0.00038	0.00012	0.00002	0.00008	0.00023	0.00019
Female age 18–34	0.20764	0.06832	0.20395	0.04478	0.13298	0.10383
No. health cond.	0.11465	0.01629	0.15474	0.00885	0.08475	0.01728
AFCAM enrolled	-0.42700	0.76411	0.13526	0.47626	-0.03102	0.41320
NAVCAM enrolled	0.56900	0.69206	-0.70287	0.30193	-0.40251	0.71260
CRI enrolled	-0.01388	0.12824	0.13721	0.07887	0.15682	0.12183
AFCAM—ret.	0.03546	0.79898	0.06705	0.51654	—	—
NAVYCAM—ret.	-0.10938	0.82494	0.53868	0.41121	—	—
CRI—ret.	0.11587	0.16672	-0.04895	0.10996	0.08657	0.06947
Army MTF	-0.17098	0.04455	0.07056	0.02955	-0.04458	0.07687
Navy MTF	-0.31971	0.04642	0.03562	0.03247	0.15398	0.09270
log(MTF beds/pop.)	0.10688	0.06731	0.12957	0.03920	0.10501	0.11383
log(beds/pop.)—ret.	0.31857	0.07645	0.01390	0.04886	0.20551	0.16561
log(MTF MDs/bed)	0.26271	0.11502	0.22326	0.06945	0.04664	0.22280
log(MDs/bed)—ret.	0.23662	0.13910	-0.00044	0.09814	0.00444	0.02679
Income—ret.	-0.06318	0.01788	0.03144	0.01174	-0.05099	0.02303
Health cond.—ret.	-0.01259	0.01881	-0.03923	0.01145		

Table C.2
MTF Use for CHAMPUS–Eligible Children in Catchment Areas

Variable	Probability of Visits>0		No. Visits if Visits>0		Probability: Hosp. Nights>0	
	Coefficient	Stand. Error	Coefficient	Stand. Error	Coefficient	Stand. Error
Intercept	0.28965	0.12309	1.06130	0.06818	-0.21093	0.17730
Retired	0.24234	0.16564	-0.23645	0.10759	-0.33170	0.17584
Officer	0.19114	0.08501	-0.06832	0.04633	—	—
Not MTF service	0.01886	0.07056	0.00873	0.03933	-0.01257	0.11504
Employed	-0.14548	0.06011	0.01395	0.03452	0.18296	0.09499
Family income	0.00789	0.02114	-0.00344	0.01161	-0.04828	0.02628
Family size	0.02614	0.02076	-0.02746	0.01229	-0.03276	0.03493
Age	-0.01663	0.01845	-0.05008	0.01045	-0.28567	0.02824
Age squared	-0.00026	0.00107	0.00156	0.00060	0.01252	0.00177
No. health cond.	0.35513	0.02712	0.27240	0.01259	0.06190	0.03281
AFCAM enrolled	-0.30640	0.54436	-0.03155	0.31580	-0.59270	1.07884
NAVCAM enrolled	-0.37034	0.53916	-0.01182	0.31777	0.02828	0.88608
CRI enrolled	-0.00832	0.10392	-0.15169	0.05479	0.04358	0.15086
AFCAM—ret.	0.69934	1.05825	0.82536	0.60264	—	—
NAVYCAM—ret.	0.56979	1.34909	-0.06042	0.81203	—	—
CRI—ret.	0.02785	0.27382	0.38646	0.18622	—	—
Army MTF	-0.20227	0.06514	0.00424	0.03470	-0.25923	0.09487
Navy MTF	-0.24879	0.06849	-0.01405	0.03716	-0.52123	0.11364
log(MTF beds/pop.)	0.28134	0.06096	0.06344	0.03187	0.45055	0.08921
log(beds/pop.—ret.	0.40827	0.11854	0.11694	0.05921	-0.47187	0.25481
log(MTF MDs/bed)	0.53372	0.10701	0.57225	0.15142	0.45089	0.17268
log(MDs/bed)—ret.	0.16338	0.22540	0.11115	0.07389	-0.35571	0.50106
Income—ret.	-0.03657	0.02937	0.05470	0.01766	—	—
Health cond.—ret.	-0.29217	0.04298	0.04276	0.03277	—	—

108

Table C.3

MTF Use for Medicare Eligibles in Catchment Areas

Variable	Probability of Visits>0		No. Visits if Visits>0		Probability: Hosp. Nights>0	
	Coefficient	Stand. Error	Coefficient	Stand. Error	Coefficient	Stand. Error
Intercept	0.72758	0.36728	0.04210	0.27968	-3.01164	0.60249
Officer	0.12264	0.07027	-0.25667	0.05062	-0.28850	0.11791
Female	-0.09778	0.06112	0.08290	0.04430	-0.19876	0.09703
Not MTF service	-0.37418	0.05871	0.07692	0.04401	-0.10597	0.09720
Family income	-0.00364	0.01563	0.07402	0.01104	0.10554	0.02139
Family size	-0.11852	0.06938	-0.30716	0.05266	-0.32468	0.12907
Age	-0.01124	0.00514	0.01004	0.00396	0.01555	0.00848
No. health cond.	0.01169	0.01165	0.13082	0.00851	0.08385	0.01732
Army MTF	0.03979	0.06915	-0.12876	0.04732	-0.27268	0.10786
Navy MTF	-0.51342	0.07412	-0.03557	0.05844	-0.43881	0.12642
log(MTF beds/pop.)	0.31131	0.05263	0.042715	0.03983	0.38831	0.08259
log(MTF MDs/bed)	-0.05662	0.10515	0.05221	0.08922	0.12064	0.17625

Table C.4

MTF Use in Noncatchment Areas

Variable	Probability of Visits>0		No. Visits if Visits>0		Probability: Hosp. Nights>0	
	Coefficient	Stand. Error	Coefficient	Stand. Error	Coefficient	Stand. Error
Intercept	-0.32341	0.20290	1.75087	0.16154	-1.23268	0.39660
Retired	-0.59340	0.17697	0.19601	0.15228	-0.58411	0.38341
Retired female	0.14021	0.06394	-0.01608	0.06280	-0.34453	0.17963
Medicare eligible	0.24189	0.13345	0.36487	0.13563	0.16996	0.32541
Officer	-0.06476	0.07849	-0.16151	0.07019	—	—
Employed	-0.10904	0.06811	-0.12690	0.05943	-0.03619	0.17105
Family income	-0.00534	0.03942	0.00989	0.02983	0.03453	0.06145
Family size	-0.04354	0.02344	-0.13819	0.02231	-0.10023	0.06269
Age	0.00761	0.00740	-0.01456	0.00647	-0.00290	0.01592
Age squared	-0.00014	0.00010	0.00005	0.00008	0.00003	0.00022
Female age 18–34	0.18497	0.11839	-0.18303	0.08973	0.08115	0.26214
No. health cond.	0.11945	0.04716	0.19904	0.03457	-0.06863	0.09819
Age—child	0.09128	0.03655	-0.07166	0.02998	0.02879	0.08494
Age squared—child	-0.00643	0.00236	0.00416	0.00194	-0.00404	0.00632
Health cond.—child	0.03236	0.06065	-0.00791	0.04850	0.03798	0.13912
Income—ret.	0.00296	0.03978	-0.00934	0.03089	-0.10791	0.07633
Health cond.—ret.	-0.09876	0.04788	-0.10840	0.03598	0.10351	0.10151
Mil. clinic area	0.47009	0.09457	-0.18864	0.06330	-0.12556	0.19912

Table C.5

CHAMPUS Use, Catchment, Active-Duty Families

Variable	Probability of Visits>0		No. Visits if Visits>0		Probability: Hosp. Nights>0	
	Coefficient	Stand. Error	Coefficient	Stand. Error	Coefficient	Stand. Error
Intercept	-1.80957	0.24327	-0.02561	0.33233	-2.28821	0.34135
Officer	0.14866	0.05034	0.19925	0.06168	0.09770	0.08657
Employed	0.03500	0.03538	0.10465	0.04392	-0.17378	0.06426
Family income	0.02293	0.01174	0.00101	0.01473	-0.03742	0.02134
Family size	0.09117	0.01209	0.09690	0.01568	0.04673	0.01969
Family age	0.03968	0.01511	0.02776	0.02073	0.00234	0.02088
Family age squared	-0.00055	0.00023	-0.00031	0.00031	0.00001	0.00031
Family health	0.10892	0.01407	0.08791	0.01729	0.10373	0.02250
Child < age 1	0.09826	0.04700	-0.10121	0.05757	0.91366	0.05997
AFCAM	-0.33482	0.27757	-0.00740	0.40703	-0.04177	0.46498
AFCAM enrolled	0.66900	0.42199	0.25429	0.54373	-0.00533	0.74979
NAVCAM	0.12691	0.11968	-0.04720	0.13483	0.39208	0.16133
NAVCAM enrolled	0.69471	0.34496	0.10456	0.30190	-0.12048	0.44885
CRI	-0.16270	0.04820	0.13883	0.06402	-0.45187	0.09929
CRI enrolled	0.72367	0.07194	0.30954	0.08090	0.65689	0.12209
Army MTF	-0.01575	0.03856	0.02248	0.04967	0.05665	0.06697
Navy MTF	0.38966	0.04404	0.26802	0.05250	0.33064	0.07172
log(MTF beds/pop)	-0.24586	0.03323	-0.08407	0.04105	-0.36669	0.05517
log(MTF MDs/bed)	-0.21993	0.05818	-0.14528	0.06319	-0.31301	0.08654
log(Civ beds/pop)	0.00817	0.00556	-0.00198	0.00706	0.00957	0.00901
log(Civ MDs/pop)	-0.03760	0.01889	0.04959	0.02493	0.02439	0.03149

Table C.6

CHAMPUS Use, Catchment, Retiree Families

Variable	Probability of Visits>0		No. Visits if Visits>0		Probability: Hosp. Nights>0	
	Coefficient	Stand. Error	Coefficient	Stand. Error	Coefficient	Stand. Error
Intercept	-2.18029	0.32507	1.17683	0.53112	-3.37253	0.80145
Officer	0.20305	0.06087	0.17601	0.06954	-0.01209	0.11250
Employed	-0.14456	0.04850	0.02559	0.05633	-0.05814	0.08638
Family income	0.03656	0.00962	0.04881	0.01106	0.01491	0.01738
Family size	0.20372	0.02046	0.03237	0.02404	0.08467	0.03486
Family age	0.02782	0.01384	-0.02101	0.02201	0.02527	0.03314
Family age squared	-0.00015	0.00015	0.00021	0.00023	-0.00015	0.00035
Family health	0.12729	0.02058	0.18126	0.02417	0.20562	0.03675
Child < age 1	-0.03094	0.30121	-0.32266	0.34014	0.31911	0.42333
AFCAM	0.01478	0.20958	0.16272	0.26268	-0.10581	0.41764
AFCAM enrolled	0.61949	0.32839	-0.19545	0.35733	0.25441	0.57344
NAVCAM	0.11664	0.20725	0.06985	0.23448	-0.16052	0.46020
NAVCAM enrolled	0.25517	0.47846	0.07408	0.49271	0.44319	0.81961
CRI	-0.40983	0.07148	0.08842	0.09576	-0.28036	0.15216
CRI enrolled	1.46073	0.14073	0.38246	0.12862	0.71072	0.20265
Army MTF	-0.02048	0.05382	-0.02016	0.06885	0.00888	0.09728
Navy MTF	0.37087	0.06030	0.28204	0.06947	0.03504	0.10835
log(MTF beds/pop)	-0.25689	0.04036	-0.20163	0.05081	-0.27341	0.07650
log(MTF MDs/bed)	-0.28787	0.07899	-0.13437	0.08823	-0.19472	0.13489
log(Civ beds/pop)	0.01561	0.00712	0.00576	0.00779	0.00641	0.01224
log(Civ MDs/pop)	-0.13220	0.02946	-0.02951	0.03539	-0.09449	0.05546

112

Table C.7

CHAMPUS Use, Noncatchment, All

Variable	Probability of Visits>0		No. Visits if Visits>0		Probability: Hosp. Nights>0	
	Coefficient	Stand. Error	Coefficient	Stand. Error	Coefficient	Stand. Error
Intercept	-1.14600	0.29514	0.34161	0.31405	-2.30383	0.50472
Officer	0.22159	0.07625	0.46085	0.07135	0.46731	0.11246
Employed	0.25151	0.05545	-0.05116	0.05467	0.12480	0.08671
Family income	-0.07356	0.03645	-0.02653	0.03710	-0.18030	0.05662
Income—ret.	0.07420	0.03640	0.02593	0.03702	0.09075	0.05711
Family size	0.12775	0.02200	0.11862	0.02120	0.05229	0.02886
Family age	0.02305	0.01430	0.00784	0.01560	0.04877	0.02551
Family age squared	-0.00010	0.00016	0.00001	0.00017	-0.00045	0.00028
Family health	0.14595	0.02238	0.15014	0.02146	0.10954	0.03392
Child < age 1	0.71504	0.13801	0.28813	0.10665	0.82126	0.14554
Mil. clinic area	0.03018	0.08706	0.06441	0.08516	-0.07399	0.12841
Retired	-0.53955	0.15230	0.14463	0.15988	-0.74090	0.23426
log(Civ beds/pop)	0.00965	0.00815	-0.01080	0.00748	0.01803	0.01114
log(Civ MDs/pop)	-0.08315	0.02438	0.08284	0.02512	-0.10270	0.04140

Table C.8

CHAMPUS Costs, Catchment, Active-Duty Families

Variable	Probability of Costs > 0		Costs if Costs > 0	
	Coefficient	Stand. Error	Coefficient	Stand. Error
Intercept	−1.00579	0.20000	4.12380	0.33997
Officer	0.09952	0.04929	0.13489	0.08546
Employed	0.00776	0.03437	−0.08887	0.06016
Family income	-0.01176	0.01145	−0.02137	0.02068
Family size	0.11950	0.01172	0.11241	0.02122
Family age	0.02821	0.01214	0.02340	0.02029
Family age squared	−0.00033	0.00018	−0.00029	0.00029
Family health	0.09397	0.01379	0.15762	0.02316
Child < age 1	0.41912	0.04736	0.73859	0.07320
AFCAM	−0.57718	0.25555	0.19389	0.54190
AFCAM enrolled	0.05293	0.40750	0.31381	0.76898
NAVCAM	0.04284	0.12043	0.10584	0.20516
NAVCAM enrolled	0.92930	0.39493	−0.34293	0.46320
CRI	−0.44949	0.04636	0.05004	0.09249
CRI enrolled	0.76747	0.07179	0.66889	0.12244
Army MTF	−0.06899	0.03724	0.09321	0.06340
Navy MTF	−0.01056	0.04355	0.59551	0.07413
log(MTF beds/pop)	−0.01838	0.03205	−0.41641	0.05321
log(MTF MDs/bed)	−0.12588	0.05728	−0.28116	0.09329
log(Civ beds/pop)	0.00270	0.00548	0.00415	0.00897
log(Civ MDs/pop)	−0.05010	0.01825	0.03031	0.03431

Table C.9

CHAMPUS Costs, Catchment, Retiree Families

Variable	Probability of Costs > 0		Costs if Costs > 0	
	Coefficient	Stand. Error	Coefficient	Stand. Error
Intercept	−2.43217	0.34521	6.44535	0.79919
Officer	0.08010	0.06085	0.28092	0.09862
Employed	−0.02928	0.04801	−0.07550	0.07772
Family income	0.02966	0.00953	−0.00538	0.01546
Family size	0.19990	0.02057	0.08897	0.03362
Family age	0.04537	0.01467	−0.07832	0.03275
Family age squared	−0.00030	0.00016	0.00089	0.00034
Family health	0.15487	0.02035	0.21728	0.03419
Child < age 1	0.53304	0.32964	−0.45132	0.41763
AFCAM	−0.29374	0.20866	0.03825	0.40705
AFCAM enrolled	1.08929	0.35003	−0.58368	0.52785
NAVCAM	−0.00851	0.20765	−0.36452	0.35221
NAVCAM enrolled	0.42034	0.48689	0.09331	0.71458
CRI	−0.71872	0.07210	0.42553	0.15467
CRI enrolled	1.46532	0.13627	0.46986	0.20497
Army MTF	0.07995	0.05265	−0.14726	0.09057
Navy MTF	0.14767	0.05999	0.32901	0.10209
log(MTF beds/pop)	−0.07058	0.03942	−0.21954	0.06743
log(MTF MDs/bed)	−0.13848	0.07842	−0.20321	0.12682
log(Civ beds/pop)	0.01344	0.00702	0.00177	0.01123
log(Civ MDs/pop)	−0.13601	0.02887	−0.08612	0.04919

Table C.10

CHAMPUS Costs, Noncatchment, All

Variable	Probability of Costs > 0		Costs if Costs > 0	
	Coefficient	Stand. Error	Coefficient	Stand. Error
Intercept	−1.12812	0.30039	3.71696	0.50140
Officer	0.25997	0.07670	0.55198	0.11739
Employed	0.26458	0.05609	−0.31644	0.08996
Family Income	−0.10460	0.03708	−0.05719	0.05689
Income—ret.	0.11307	0.03708	−0.00886	0.05706
Family size	0.13889	0.02246	0.14770	0.03385
Family age	0.02484	0.01455	0.05462	0.02514
Family age squared	−0.00007	0.00016	−0.00063	0.00028
Family health	0.18720	0.02281	0.24952	0.03588
Child < age 1	0.95784	0.15076	0.82101	0.16603
Mil. clinic area	0.13406	0.08875	0.09744	0.13134
Retired	−0.98735	0.15598	0.33623	0.25134
log(Civ beds/pop)	0.00115	0.00821	0.01788	0.01279
log(Civ MDs/pop)	−0.08214	0.02471	0.04472	0.04269

Table C.11

Weighted Means and Standard Deviations for Variables in MTF Regressions

Variable	Catchment Areas — CHAMPUS-Eligible Adults		Catchment Areas — Children		Catchment Areas — Medicare Eligibles		Non-Catchment Areas — All Beneficiaries	
	Mean	Std. Dev.	Mean	Std. Dev.	Mean	Std. Dev.	Mean	Std. Dev.
Any visits	0.5288	0.4984	0.6455	0.4725	0.4122	0.4830	0.2418	0.4216
log (visits)	1.1710	0.7306	1.0748	0.7045	1.2592	0.6878	1.1481	0.6569
Any inpatient	0.0565	0.2309	0.0653	0.2472	0.0543	0.2267	0.0158	0.1246
Retired	0.6699	0.4703	0.2579	0.4376			0.8225	0.3892
Retired female	0.3300	0.4703			0.5277	0.4905	0.4264	0.4946
Medicare							0.1884	0.3911
Officer	0.2040	0.4030	0.1829	0.3866	0.4324	0.4955	0.2174	0.4125
Not MTF service	0.2582	0.4377	0.1756	0.3805	0.3907	0.4880		
Employed	0.4752	0.4982	0.2971	0.4570			0.3223	0.4674
Family income grp.	4.3089	0.0175	3.3842	1.9513	3.3735	2.1256	3.6011	2.3219
Family size	3.0152	1.4301	4.1749	1.4017	0.0162	0.0223	2.7910	1.5602
Single					0.3481	0.4765		
Age	43.2124	14.0893	7.8237	5.0853	72.3642	5.9810	44.1336	23.1304
Female age 18–34	0.2447	0.4289					0.0770	0.2626
No. conditions	2.2936	2.2447	1.4737	1.4352	3.1355	2.3572	2.3699	2.2792
AFCAM enrolled	0.0059	0.0763	0.0027	0.0523				
NAVCAM enrolled	0.0025	0.0498	0.0020	0.0448				
CRI enrolled	0.0481	0.2141	0.0678	0.2514				
AFCAM—ret.	0.0054	0.0733	0.0012	0.0339				
NAVYCAM—ret.	0.0016	0.0394	0.0004	0.0191				
CRI—ret.	0.0277	0.1641	0.0124	0.1108				
Army MTF	0.3820	0.4859	0.4193	0.4935	0.3489	0.4767		
Navy MTF	0.2749	0.4465	0.2847	0.4513	0.3064	0.4611		
log(MTF beds/pop)	0.4143	0.7179	0.4393	0.6855	0.4219	0.7379		
log(beds/pop)—ret.	0.2707	0.6548	0.0988	0.4325				
log(MTF MDs/bed)	-0.3340	0.3694	-0.3321	0.3627	-0.3254	0.3899		
log(MDs/bed)—ret.	-0.2301	0.3497	-0.0875	0.2474				
Area w/ clinic							0.0920	0.2891
Income—ret.	3.1424	3.2137	0.9387	2.0109			3.0444	2.6253
Health cond.—chld							0.3230	0.8569
Health cond.—ret.	1.6180	2.2030	0.4481	0.4481	0	0	0000000	0000000

Table C.12

Weighted Means and Standard Deviations for Variables in CHAMPUS Regressions

| | Catchment Areas | | | | Non-Catchment Areas | |
| | Active-Duty Families | | Retired Families | | All Families | |
Variable	Mean	Std. Dev.	Mean	Std. Dev.	Mean	Std. Dev.
Any visits	0.3591	0.4798	0.4053	0.4910	0.6034	0.48930
log (visits)	1.4337	1.0144	1.6550	1.0401	1.7806	1.07290
Any inpatient	0.0622	0.2415	0.0391	0.1939	0.1091	0.31180
Any govt. costs	0.5361	0.4987	0.4916	0.5000	0.6099	0.48790
log (govt. costs)	5.6712	1.7114	5.6603	1.5787	6.2287	1.82560
Any costs	0.5726	0.4947	0.5347	0.4989	0.6721	0.46950
log(total costs)	5.8606	1.6432	6.1560	1.5968	6.5308	1.69010
Officer	0.1844	0.3878	0.1968	0.3976	0.2771	0.4476
Employed	0.2755	0.4468	0.5120	0.4999	0.3186	0.4660
Family income catg.	3.2464	1.8982	4.5681	2.7431	3.8776	2.2979
Family income—ret.					1.6340	2.6694
Family size	3.6008	1.3148	2.5048	1.1885	3.1405	1.3636
Family age	30.9373	7.3634	50.5150	9.7165	40.1596	12.7471
Family health	2.3458	1.0827	2.8082	1.0816	2.5014	1.1391
Child < age 1	0.1242	0.3299	0.0050	0.0702	0.0454	0.2081
AFCAM	0.0052	0.0719	0.0167	0.1282		
AFCAM enrolled	0.0019	0.0438	0.0063	0.0792		
NAVCAM	0.0170	0.1295	0.0131	0.1137		
NAVCAM enrolled	0.0020	0.0449	0.0022	0.0472		
CRI	0.1931	0.3948	0.1696	0.3753		
CRI enrolled	0.0651	0.2467	0.0399	0.1958		
Army MTF	0.4329	0.4955	0.3598	0.4800		
Navy MTF	0.2978	0.4673	0.2704	0.4442		
log(MTF beds/pop)	0.4464	0.6244	0.3923	0.7517		
log(MTF MDs/bed)	-0.3240	0.3509	-0.3343	0.3756		
Area w/ clinic					0.2462	0.4309
Retired family					0.3954	0.4890
Civ beds/pop	4.4272	3.2950	4.3828	3.6593	5.2418	3.2778
Civ MDs/pop	1.6427	0.9692	1.7120	0.8801	1.9117	1.2928

D. Adjustments to MTF Utilization Estimates for Costing by IDA

The demand analysis yielded estimates of per-capita MTF visits and the fraction of beneficiaries hospitalized. Before these estimates could be sent to IDA for costing, we needed to modify them in four ways:

1. Adjust the per-capita estimates derived from the survey to make them compatible with MEPRS workload data,

2. Multiply by the number of beneficiaries to get total MTF workloads for the beneficiaries studied,

3. Add the workloads for active-duty personnel and "other beneficiaries," and the workloads in the United States for overseas beneficiaries, and

4. Allocate the total workload to individual MTFs.

The third step is self-explanatory, so this appendix focuses on the other three steps.

Adjusting to MEPRS Workload Levels

An adjustment was necessary because all of our predictions of utilization are based upon the survey (the only source of utilization outside of the MTFs and CHAMPUS), while all of the estimates for costing the MTFs are based upon workload derived from the accounting systems (specifically MEPRS).

The method we used to determine the adjustment factors was simple. First, we used the demand regressions (described in Section 5 and Appendix C) to predict the average number of visits and the fraction of beneficiaries hospitalized for each type of beneficiary under the 1992 conditions. The beneficiary groups were: active-duty dependents; retirees under age 65; retirees' dependents, survivors, and their dependents under age 65; and all beneficiaries 65 and older. We then calculated a second set of per-capita utilization figures—in this case, average number of visits and admissions—by dividing the utilization reported in MEPRS by the DEERS-based population estimates described below. For each beneficiary group, the adjustment factors equaled the MEPRS/DEERS utilization estimates divided by the utilization estimates predicted from the regressions. We

118

examined all areas in the United States, excluding only overseas hospitalizations and outpatient visits.

Factors for Outpatient Care

The outpatient visit adjustment factors are shown in Table D.1. These numbers are what the survey-derived estimates of outpatient visits must be multiplied by to produce the per-capita number of MEPRS outpatient visits for each of these types of beneficiary. These factors include: (1) an adjustment for the windsorized survey data (at 10), (2) downward bias in the survey data because of imperfect recall, and (3) the inclusion of more types of patient encounters in MEPRS.

Table D.1

Outpatient Adjustment Factors

Active-Duty Dependents	Retirees Under 65	Retired Dependents/ Survivors Under 65	Beneficiaries 65 and Over
1.80	2.07	1.33	1.48

Since IDA's analysis showed that outpatient costs are higher in Navy MTFs, we looked to see whether the adjustment factors differed by service. Table D.2 compares the factors for outpatient visits by service for all nonoverlapping catchment areas. The Navy factors are lower, suggesting that there may be some modest difference in the accounting procedures among the services.

We also looked for other possible differences (e.g., whether medical centers varied consistently one way or another), but we did not find any consistent patterns.

Table D.2

Service Differences in Outpatient Exchange Factors

Service	Exchange Factor
Army	1.87
Air Force	1.61
Navy	1.29

Factors for Inpatient Care

The raw inpatient exchange factors are shown in Table D.3. These numbers are what the survey-derived estimates of the average probabilities of being hospitalized must be multiplied by to produce the per-capita number of MEPRS inpatient admissions for each beneficiary group. These multipliers include: (1) same-day hospitalizations—included in MEPRS but not in the data used in the regressions, and (2) the average number of hospitalizations per person hospitalized.

Table D.3

Inpatient Exchange Factors

Active-Duty Dependents	Retirees Under 65	Retired Dependents/ Survivors Under 65	Beneficiaries 65 and Over
1.33	1.25	1.21	1.25

Estimating the Number of Beneficiaries

Table D.4 compares the estimates of FY92 beneficiary populations in the official DEERS data, our adjusted figures for FY92, and a late-90s estimate of the beneficiary populations, assuming the closing of all MTFs affected through BRAC 3 and a reduction in the DoD population consistent with DoD's recently completed "Bottom-Up Review."

The short-record DEERS record that is archived and released for analysis records the sponsor's zip code for all active-duty dependents. This ignores the fact that many active-duty members are sent overseas each year for unaccompanied duty, their family often returning to live with relatives in noncatchment areas. In FY90, this assumption increases the number of active-duty dependents counted as being overseas by some 300,000, with nearly the same reduction in the noncatchment areas.[1] We used a modified version of the short record that provides actual locations for active-duty dependents. We adjusted these data at the individual zip-code level because of the following:

---

[1]This problem is related to the change in counting active duty dependents in FY92 that is noted above.

- A distance check of the zip codes around military hospitals showed that several zip codes with large numbers of beneficiaries were well within 40 miles of the hospital, and yet treated in DEERS as though these areas were noncatchment areas. An examination of the zip codes with the largest military populations showed that they had been introduced since 1990, and thus were omitted from the catchment-area directory of zip codes. We have corrected the more obvious of these problems, transferring roughly 1,000 active-duty personnel, 7,000 active-duty dependents, and 11,000 retired and other beneficiaries from noncatchment to catchment areas.

- While the year-end DEERS theoretically reports beneficiary location on September 30th of the given year, it is actually compiled some months thereafter, reflecting the movement of any beneficiaries who have reported to new locations. However, because DEERS also includes information on personnel recruited but not yet inducted into the military, the DEERS data must be handled with a strict date of effectiveness, which we have chosen to

Table D.4

Beneficiary Populations

Type of Beneficiary	Location	FY92 DEERS	Adjusted FY92 DEERS	Late-90s Estimate
Active duty	Catchment	1,350,489	1,383,956	1,117,418
Active-duty dependent	Catchment	1,930,885	1,958,358	1,520,383
Nat'l. Guard/Reserve	Catchment	110,211	113,092	66,166
NG/Reserve dependent	Catchment	152,503	153,049	92,770
Retired < 65	Catchment	711,217	714,178	579,748
Retired 65+	Catchment	318,331	319,738	293,190
Other < 65	Catchment	1,222,749	1,227,917	1,049,148
Other 65+	Catchment	310,453	311,681	289,543
Active duty	Noncatch	136,798	123,077	130,649
Active-duty dependent	Noncatch	286,837	438,061	321,419
Nat'l. Guard/Reserve	Noncatch	100,251	90,622	63,426
NG/Reserve dependent	Noncatch	96,044	95,498	86,072
Retired < 65	Noncatch	415,441	412,480	491,687
Retired 65+	Noncatch	216,177	214,770	305,303
Other < 65	Noncatch	599,737	594,569	723,702
Other 65+	Noncatch	152,246	151,018	226,213
Active duty	Overseas	307,920	307,920	182,093
Active-duty dependent	Overseas	349,332	169,078	131,594
Nat'l. Guard/Reserve	Overseas	1,469	1,469	1,787
NG/Reserve dependent	Overseas	6,799	6,799	3,822
Retired < 65	Overseas	11,125	11,125	14,828
Retired 65+	Overseas	1,468	1,468	3,820
Other < 65	Overseas	17,838	17,838	17,064
Other 65+	Overseas	892	892	3,079
Total	All	8,807,212	8,818,654	7,714,924

NOTE: Total does not include beneficiaries in unknown locations.

retain at September 30, 1992. But since the data on location is actually many months later for many individuals, training bases (such as Ft. Jackson, Great Lakes, Lackland AFB, or Parris Island) have very low counts of trainees (those of E-1 rank, both active duty and National Guard/Reserve) because many of the trainees have moved on by the time DEERS was compiled. We therefore used DoD and Army estimates of personnel in the training pipeline and actual personnel at selected bases to adjust the DEERS estimates for both active-duty personnel and active-duty dependents. For example, DEERS shows Ft. Jackson with only about 7,000 active-duty personnel at the end of FY92, whereas Army and DoD figures would suggest a number closer to 13,000 (counting National Guard and Reserve personnel, in each case). Besides the basic training facilities, we have also made population adjustments at training facilities such as Ft. Irwin, where the Army reports that the DEERS numbers of active-duty beneficiaries are only about half of the active-duty population, on average, at Ft. Irwin. These adjustments cause a net increase in active-duty and Guard/Reserve personnel and their dependents in catchment areas, and a decrease in noncatchment areas.

- The 1992 DEERS counts show a substantial increase in the number of overseas active-duty dependents compared with previous years, and an offsetting decline in active-duty dependents in the United States (especially in noncatchment areas). The change is reportedly an accounting change, whereby dependents lacking a recent address update are now located at the unit address of their sponsor. DEERS thus considers many dependents of sponsors on overseas, unaccompanied tours to be overseas as well. Because this change appears wrong, we have adjusted the active-duty dependent numbers to more closely reflect the pattern of location in previous years, shifting about 180,000 active-duty dependents back to the United States (mostly to noncatchment areas).

To project beneficiaries for the late 1990s, we began with the FY92 DEERS data and an aggregate RAPS (Resource Analysis and Planning System) estimate of beneficiaries by catchment area. We adjusted these to reflect the results of BRAC 3 and the problem with the training bases noted above. The result is a zip-code-level projection of the beneficiary population for the late 1990s, which can be aggregated to catchment area or grand total levels (the latter shown in Table D.3 above).

Our explorations uncovered several problems in using the DEERS data that either did not affect the beneficiary groups we studied or could not be corrected:

- Because military personnel move fairly often, are promoted regularly, add dependents, and so forth, DEERS is almost always somewhat out-of-date. Civilian health plans have similar problems, as individuals move and/or change employers. HMOs, which must plan using per-capita information by location, go to considerable effort to update addresses (e.g., checking them at each encounter with the beneficiary).

- Some advanced education locations like the Army War College at Carlisle Barracks apparently only have their staff properly located in DEERS; their students appear to be shown as part of a training command located elsewhere. The same is true for the many military personnel involved in detached training at various locations around the country.

- The location given for active-duty beneficiaries may be a unit address or home address. An active-duty beneficiary who lives in Northern Virginia in the Ft. Belvoir catchment area but works in Washington, D.C., in the Walter Reed catchment area, might be counted in either area (and also might get care in either area).

- In recent years, over 200,000 active-duty Navy personnel have been considered "AFLOAT," which apparently means that they are assigned to a ship. The average surface ship appears to be at sea about 40 percent of the time, and in its home port only about half of the remaining time. Therefore, many of these personnel are not, at any given time, living in their assigned catchment area.

- For FY92, DEERS lists some 230,000 Army National Guard and Reserve personnel on active duty, whereas the National Guard Bureau suggested that the number may be perhaps only a third as much. Apparently some Guard and Reserve personnel not on regular active duty are included in DEERS, and some are not.

- The definitions of catchment areas have some potential flaws. For example, there is no catchment area for Ft. Drum, which has a clinic but has arranged for its providers to treat patients in the local civilian hospital, but there is a catchment area for Newport NS, which has a similar arrangement. Catchment areas are defined for several of the U.S. Treatment Facilities (former Public Health Service hospitals). Unless many military beneficiaries use these facilities, creating these catchment areas causes an underestimate of the noncatchment population and of the catchment-area population for facilities that overlap (such as Ft. Meade).

Distributing Workload to MTFs

The workloads at the MTFs for the analytic cases are predicted for all beneficiaries living in aggregated U.S. catchment or noncatchment areas. For inpatient use, the aggregation is to type of beneficiary in either catchment or noncatchment areas. For outpatient use, the aggregation is to type of beneficiary in 10 catchment-area groups (small hospitals, medium hospitals, and medical centers for the Army, Navy, and Air Force, plus an overlapping catchment-area group), and also a non-catchment-area group. For costing, we needed to distribute the aggregate workloads to the individual MTFs and by broad specialty categories.

To make this distribution for case 1, we developed a "referral" matrix. The inpatient referral matrix was calculated from FY90 biometrics data to show the fraction of people from each catchment-area group hospitalized in that group and other groups. For example, 59 percent of retirees under 65 living in small Navy catchment areas were hospitalized in those facilities, while 25 percent were hospitalized in MTFs with overlapping catchment areas, 5 percent in Navy medical centers, and 4 percent in medium Naval hospitals. We estimated a similar matrix for outpatient referrals by comparing our predicted workloads by group with MEPRS workloads for the same groups (the latter do not report the location of people receiving outpatient care at the various MTFs). These matrices were used for case 1, but not case 2, because there was no reason to expect that the added workloads in case 2 would follow the referral patterns described in the matrices.

An example of how we used these matrices to distribute the MTF workloads predicted for case 1 may be helpful. If Air Force medical centers had 1,000,000 outpatient visits by active-duty dependents in FY90, and Scott AFB had 150,000 of these, then we allocated to Scott 15 percent of the case 1 visits we predicted for Air Force medical centers.

For case 2, we used regression analysis to estimate MTF production functions that we could use to predict the increase in each MTF's inpatient and outpatient workloads that would result from an increase in operating beds and staffing. We then allocated the increase in predicted workloads from case 1 to case 2 in proportion to the workload increase that we predicted from the production function. For example, if we predicted 120,000 added visits at Scott AFB and a total increase at all MTFs of 6,000,000 extra visits, then if the total number of active-duty-dependent visits increased by 1,000,000 in case 2, Scott would receive 50,000 of these added visits.

Finally, we allocated the workloads by specialty category—medical, obstetrics and gynecology, pediatrics, psychiatry, and surgery—according to the historical specialty distribution at each MTF. For example, if the hospital at Scott AFB had 12 percent of its outpatient workload in surgery in FY90 and total outpatient visits increased from 300,000 in case 1 to 350,000 in case 2, then Scott would have 42,000 visits in surgery.

E. Analyses to Predict MTF Utilization and Civilian Costs for Cases 3 and 4

This appendix gives more detailed descriptions of the analyses conducted to study cases 3 and 4, including: (1) the regression models for predicting choice of health plan; (2) the simulation model for simulating the costs of civilian fee-for-service plans; (3) a summary of the effects of cost sharing on health care costs and outcomes measured in the Health Insurance Experiment, whose results we relied on in several of the analyses; and (4) the regressions estimated to predict MTF utilization for case 4.

Choice of Health Care Plan

The simulation of health-plan choices is based on a sequential decisionmaking model. Families are assumed to choose whether to enroll in the military health plan or to receive their care through the civilian health care system. Conditional on the choice of the civilian system, families select whether to enroll in an HMO or a fee-for-service health care plan. This appendix describes the behavioral models in our choice simulation and the simulation methods.

Choice Between the Military and Civilian Health Care System

The data for the model of health care system choice come from the 1992 DoD Health Care Survey described in Section 3. Participants in the survey were presented with two hypothetical alternatives to their existing military health plan.[1] Both alternatives cover the same broad scope of services as the CHAMPUS program with the added benefit of preventive exams and routine eye care. In both plans, the only cost sharing is a $5-per-visit charge for outpatient visits. One plan is a military HMO that would require patients to receive all care from the military treatment facility. The other plan was described as a civilian health maintenance organization; however, we interpret the responses to this plan as evidencing a preference for civilian care over the current mixed system. For each of these plans, survey respondents were asked to indicate whether they would join the new plan instead of their current military plan if the new plan

---

[1]The relevant questions from the survey instrument are reproduced at the end of this appendix.

charged a premium of $75 per month, a premium of $50 per month, or no premium.

We estimate the parameters of the enrollment choice model by drawing on expected utility theory. A family will prefer one of the hypothetical plans presented in the survey to their current coverage if the expected utility of the hypothetical plan exceeds the expected utility of the current plan, i.e., if

$$EU(New\ Option) - EU(Current\ Plan) > 0. \qquad (1)$$

We assume that this difference, which we will denote as I^*, is a linear function of characteristics of the family (x) and plan (p) and is given by :

$$I^* = xA + pB + u, \qquad (2)$$

where u is a stochastic term. Let $y = 1$ if the family reports that it would purchase the new option; we have:

$$\Pr(y = 1) = \Pr(I^* > 0) = \Pr(xA + pB + u > 0).$$

If the u is from a normal distribution, then we can estimate the parameters A and B using probit regression. The family characteristics (x) in the regression model include: demographic characteristics of the sponsor; whether the family has insurance in addition to the military coverage; length of residence in the area; family size; family income; health status and expected health care use; whether the family's usual source of care is the military or civilian system; service; and characteristics of the military health-supply system in the residence area. The characteristics of the plan are whether it is a military or civilian option and the premium cost to enroll. Interactions between family characteristics and the type of alternative plan are included in the model to detect differences in preferences for the military and civilian system among different subgroups. We fit separate models for three subgroups of families: dependents of active-duty military; retirees under age 65; and retirees age 65 and older.

Because each family was asked to report about six different plans (the military HMO at three premium quotes and the all-civilian option at three premium quotes), we have multiple observations on the dependent variable for each family. Our estimation sample included 89,281 responses about preferences for hypothetical plans. We correct inference statistics for the intrafamily correlation resulting from these multiple observations using available software for the probit based on Huber's (1967) approach for nonparametric estimates.

The results of our estimation models are given in Tables E.1–E.3 for dependents of active-duty personnel, for retirees under age 65, and for older retirees, respectively. Each table reports the effect of a change in the explanatory variable on the probability of choosing the military HMO in preference to CHAMPUS or other military plan in which the family is enrolled and the effect on the probability of choosing the new civilian plan in preference to CHAMPUS; the changes in probability are evaluated at the mean probability for the group.

Table E.1

Effects of Family and Plan Characteristics on Preference for Hypothetical Plans: Dependents of Active-Duty Personnel

Characteristic	Civilian Plan	Military Plan	Significant Difference
Demographic and economic characteristics			
Sponsor characteristics			
Male	2.4*	–2.4	*
White	–1.5*	–5.4*	*
Education[a]			
Some college/college grad.	0.2	–3.1*	*
Post college	–1.5	–6.0*	*
Age (10% increase)	0.1	1.1*	*
Family has other insurance	2.2*	0.2	*
At current location over 1 year	–0.3	–1.4	
Family size			
Number eligible adults	0.1	2.4*	*
Number eligible children	–0.4	–0.8*	
Income (10% change)	0.2*	0.1	*
Health characteristics			
Sickest member health[b]			
Good	1.8*	0.6	*
Fair	1.9*	-0.4	*
Poor	2.6	-2.7	*
Expected hospitalization if MTF usual source	–0.2	1.5	
Expected hospitalization if civilian usual source	2.1	6.0*	
Expected doctor visits if MTF usual source	–0.1	–0.3*	*
Expected doctor visits if civilian usual source	–0.2*	–0.6*	*
Usually use military facility	–4.0*	2.6*	*
Service[c]			
Navy	0.4	–5.3*	*
Air Force	–3.3*	–4.5*	
Marines	–2.8*	–5.3*	
MTF supply characteristics			
Operating beds/1000 population (10% increase)	–0.1*	0.0	*
Clinical FTE/operating beds (10% increase)	0.0	0.0	
Premium ($10/month increase)		–7.3*	

[a]High school or less category omitted .
[b]Excellent or very good category omitted .
[c]Army category omitted.
*Significant at p = 0.05.

Table E.2

Effects of Family and Plan Characteristics on Preference for Hypothetical Plans: Retirees Under Age 65

Characteristic	Change in Probability of Preferring New Plan to CHAMPUS with Change in Characteristic		
	Civilian Plan	Military Plan	Significant Difference
Demographic and economic characteristics			
Sponsor characteristics			
Male	4.5*	2.1	
White	0.5	–6.5*	*
Education[a]			
Some college/college grad.	–0.0	–0.0	
Post college	–0.1	–1.7	
Age (10% increase)	0.2	2.9*	*
Family has other insurance	4.0*	2.9*	*
At current location over 1 year	–1.7	–2.8	
Family size			
Number eligible adults	–0.1	0.9	
Number eligible children	0.6	0.7	
Income (10% change)	0.2*	–0.0	*
Health characteristics			
Sickest member health[b]			
Good	0.5	0.1	
Fair	–0.5	–0.1	
Poor	–4.3*	–3.5	
Expected hospitalization if MTF usual source	1.0	3.6*	
Expected hospitalization if civilian usual source	0.7	2.5	
Expected doctor visits if MTF usual source	–0.2*	–0.4*	
Expected doctor visits if civilian usual source	–0.2*	–0.6*	
Usually use military facility	–5.8*	6.1*	*
Service[c]			
Navy	0.3	–2.4	
Air Force	–0.6	–1.3	
Marines	–0.6	–11.9*	*
MTF supply characteristics			
Operating beds/1000 population (10% increase)	0.0	0.2	
Clinical FTE/operating beds (10% increase)	0.0	0.0	
Premium ($10/month increase)		–5.5*	

[a]High school or less category omitted .
[b]Excellent or very good category omitted.
[c]Army category omitted.
*Significant at p = 0.05.

Table E.3

Effects of Family and Plan Characteristics on Preference for Hypothetical Plans:
Retirees Age 65 or Older

Characteristic	Change in Probability of Preferring New Plan to CHAMPUS with Change in Characteristic		
	Civilian Plan	Military Plan	Significant Difference
Demographic and economic characteristics			
Sponsor characteristics			
Male	7.5*	6.0	
White	2.9	–7.8*	*
Education[a]			
Some college/college grad.	–0.1	0.1	
Post college	–0.7	1.6	
Age (10% increase)	–0.5	1.0	*
Family has other insurance	3.0*	3.0*	
At current location over 1 year	0.0	–0.9	
Family size			
Number eligible adults	1.8*	3.0*	
Number eligible children	–0.6	–1.0	
Income (10% change)	0.3*	–0.1	*
Health characteristics			
Sickest member health[b]			
Good	0.6	1.8	
Fair	–0.9	–0.9	
Poor	–0.4	–1.0	
Expected hospitalization if MTF usual source	2.7*	2.3	
Expected hospitalization if civilian usual source	2.9*	4.2*	
Expected doctor visits if MTF usual source	–0.4*	–0.3*	
Expected doctor visits if civilian usual source	–0.4*	–0.6*	
Usually use military facility	–7.0*	1.1	*
Service[c]			
Navy	–0.6	0.9	
Air Force	2.4*	3.8*	
Marines	–0.6	–2.9	
MTF supply characteristics			
Operating beds/1000 population (10% increase)	–0.1*	–0.0	*
Clinical FTE/operating beds (10% increase)	–0.2*	–0.1	
Premium ($10/month increase)	–5.7*		

[a]High school or less category omitted.
[b]Excellent or very good category omitted.
[c]Army category omitted.
*Significant at $p = 0.05$.

130

The parameters of the model were estimated on the basis of responses from all military personnel, including personnel living in catchment areas and those not in catchment areas. The latter were asked to respond to the questions as if they lived near an MTF.[2] We tested whether the reported preference for the different options did vary between those living in catchment areas and others and whether their response to variations in the premium differed. We did not find statistically significant differences for any of the three groups (Chi-square with 3 degrees of freedom equals 4.8 for active-duty personnel, 0.1 for retirees under age 65, and 3.9 for retirees over age 65). We also tested for a different response to the premium depending on whether the option was a military or civilian plan, and found no statistically significant differences in the three groups (t=0.7 for active-duty personnel and for retiress under age 65, t=0.6 for retirees over age 65).

To study case 4, we use our estimated model to simulate whether active-duty and retired military personnel and their families living in catchment areas would choose to enroll in a military HMO or to obtain care in the civilian system. Families in noncatchment areas are restricted to a choice among alternative civilian plans as described below. To simulate the choice of delivery system for those in catchment areas, we use Eq. 2 to predict the difference in the expected utility of a military HMO as compared with the current CHAMPUS system, $I^*(M)$, as

$$I^*(M) = xA(M) + pB + u(M),$$

and the difference in the expected utility of a civilian plan and the current system, $I^*(C)$, as

$$I^*(C) = xA(C) + pB + u(C),$$

using the parameters from the probit model and assumptions about the premium for the plans. The $u(M)$ and $u(C)$ are drawn from a bivariate normal distibution with unit variance. We estimate the correlation between the $u(M)$ and $u(C)$ using a sample of the residuals from the probit regression measured as the difference between the reported 0,1 preference response for a new plan and the predicted probability of selecting the plan. The estimated correlation beween the $u(M)$ and $u(C)$ was 0.45 for families of active-duty personnel, 0.57 for families of retirees under age 65, and 0.67 for retirees age 65 and older.

---

[2]In our simulation of case 4, however, personnel who live in a noncatchment area are assumed to select one of the civilian options; that is, they do not have a choice between the military and civilian delivery systems.

Choice Between Alternative Civilian Plans

For the second stage of our sequential decisionmaking model, we used data from the 1987 National Medical Expenditure Survey (NMES) to estimate a model of choice between civilian FFS and HMO plans. The NMES was a panel survey that was administered to a cross section of the civilian, noninstitutional population to measure health-insurance coverage, health status and health care use.

The sample for our estimation was limited to families with an insured, working family head who had a choice of health-insurance plans from his or her employer. The estimation sample included 1,508 families. We limited the sample in this way to model the FFS-HMO enrollment decision among families who had the opportunity to enroll in an HMO. Our criterion, however, imperfectly selects those families who have this opportunity. For some families who have a choice of insurance plans, the choice will be among high- and low-option FFS plans. For others, the choice may be between an FFS plan and some managed-care plan other than an HMO. However, the data available to us do not provide the information to make more accurate selections.

We used a probit regression, similar to the regression used for the military-civilian choice model, to estimate the relationship between family characteristics and the decision to enroll in an HMO instead of an FFS plan.[3] Our model results are given in Table E.4.

For families who are predicted to use the civilian sector in the first stage of the decision and for families who are not in catchment areas, we use the model estimated from the NMES data to determine whether the family enrolls in the civilian HMO or the civilian fee-for-service plan. Our sequential decision model assumes that the choice of civilian HMO is independent of whether a military plan is among the options available to the family.

While this is a strong and untestable assumption, we believe it is reasonable to assume that families' first choice is whether they want to receive care from military or civilian providers and that relative preferences among civilian alternatives are similar for military personnel living in catchment areas and those not in catchment areas.

Using the model fit with the NMES data, a family in the civilian delivery system is determined to enroll in the civilian HMO instead of the FFS plan if $\gamma X + \varepsilon > 0$, where γ is the estimated parameters of the model and ε is drawn

---

[3]We do not have details about the benefits or costs of the options that the family faces to include in our estimation model.

Table E.4

**Effects of Family Characteristics on Choice of HMO Among
Civilian Options: Results from National Medical Expenditure Survey**

Characteristic	Change in Probability of Selecting HMO for Change in Characteristic
Demographic and economic characteristics	
Primary insured characteristics	
Male	+12.0*
White	−12.5*
Education[a]	
Some college/college grad.	6.9*
Post-college	7.7*
Age (10% increase)	−0.5
Family has other insurance	−0.2
Number persons in insurance unit	
Income (10% change)	0.5
Health characteristics	
Sickest member health[b]	
Good	0.6
Fair	3.6
Poor	7.8
Hospital days past year	−0.2
Physician visits past year	−0.0

[a]High school or less category omitted.
[b]Excellent or very good category omitted.
*Significant at $p = 0.05$.

from a standard normal distribution. As we discussed in Section 6, we believe the HMO enrollments in our NMES estimation sample underestimate enrollments among families who have a choice of plan because data limitations did not allow us to identify precisely those families that were offered an HMO as an alternative. Therefore, we adjusted the fitted intercept in our probit model to result in predicted probabilities that accord with the BLS overall estimate of 35 percent enrollments.

Health Expenditures Simulation Model

To estimate costs for beneficiaries predicted to enroll in a fee-for-service civilian health plan, we used a health expenditures simulation model developed at RAND. The model predicts individual and family health-plan expenditures for fee-for-service health-insurance plans as a function of the structure of that insurance.

Health-insurance plans typically include a mix of deductibles, coinsurance rates, and upper limits on the patient's out-of-pocket expenses in a year. The price that an individual faces when making medical-care decisions may change during the course of a year from 100 percent of the charge (before the deductible is exceeded), to the coinsurance rate (a specified share of the billed charge), to zero or full coverage (when the upper limit is exceeded). Thus the plan presents the consumer with a price schedule rather than a single price.

The price that the consumer faces at any time may affect two decisions about a treatment episode. The first is the decision to begin an episode by contacting a doctor, for example, when flu symptoms are experienced or when it is time for an annual physical. An episode of treatment includes all the expenditures associated with a particular bout of illness; any individual typically has several treatment episodes during a year. Once a patient has decided to obtain care, the patient and doctor determine how much to spend on care for that episode. This decision, too, may be affected by the share of the cost the patient will have to bear.

The Health Insurance Experiment (HIE) examined the effect of price and individual characteristics on four types of medical episodes: hospitalization, outpatient chronic, outpatient acute, and well care. The results of the analyses showed that price has a significant impact on the rate at which the patient initiates episodes. For example, with 25 percent cost sharing, the rate of occurrence of ambulatory episodes is about 75 to 80 percent of the occurrence rate with no cost sharing. Initial deductibles further reduce the rate at which patients initiate episodes. The effect of price on hospital episodes is somewhat smaller than the effect of price on ambulatory episodes. Price, however, has only a small effect on the total cost of an episode; that is, it appears that cost sharing affects patients' decisions to initiate episodes but has only small effects on doctors' decisions about how to treat patients.[4] The analyses also revealed that price appears to be relatively unimportant when catastrophic illness occurs. Specifically, the rate at which "catastrophic" or very expensive hospitalizations occur was not affected by the level of patient cost sharing (Keeler et al., 1988).

The behavioral results of the HIE episode analysis have been incorporated in a stochastic simulation model that generates the occurrence of episodes for a family throughout the year depending on characteristics of the members of the family and the price facing the family (see Buchanan et al., 1991).

---

[4]This HIE result pertains only to the effects of patient cost sharing on doctors' decisions about treatment. With the growth of managed-care plans, it is possible that doctors' treatment decisions may vary with other aspects of plan design, including whether the plan requires utilization review and fee discounting. The two studies that have investigated this question (Garnick et al., 1990, and Wouters, 1990) reached different conclusions. However, both studies were limited to relatively routine types of care that were not subject to utilization review at the time and did not separate physician decisions on treatment from patient decisions to seek care.

Each family is assumed to have an underlying propensity to experience each of the four medical episode types (hospitalization, outpatient chronic, outpatient acute, and well care). The propensity to experience each episode type consists of a measured component determined by characteristics of the family and its individual members along with an unmeasured component that reflects unobserved characteristics of the family. The unmeasured component for each episode type is drawn from a gamma distribution across episode types. This reflects the finding that families who have an above-average propensity to experience hospital episodes (given the family-measured characteristics) also have an above-average propensity to experience outpatient acute and chronic episodes, and that the occurrence rates for the outpatient medical episodes are also correlated. The propensity for any family is the sum of the propensities for each family member; these individual propensities depend on the demographic and health characteristics of the individual and on economic characteristics of the family, such as income.

Given the estimated propensity to experience episodes, the model simulates the actual occurrence of episodes for a family one at a time during a year. The episodes are generated from a Poisson process. For each episode, the model determines the type of episode and the family member to whom it occurs based on the propensities for each family member to experience each episode type.

Once an episode occurs, the total expenditure for the episode is estimated. The log expenditure of the episode is randomly generated from a normal distribution, with a mean that depends on the type of episode and the characteristics of the individual experiencing it. Because the health care utilization patterns depicted in the HIE are now somewhat outdated, we have introduced an adjustment to the episode-size calculation to account for changes in the medical intensity of treatment patterns through time. These intensity parameters were derived from the Health Care Financing Administration's (HCFA's) National Expenditure Accounts.

The rate at which the family experiences episodes and, to a lesser extent, the cost of an episode depend on the effective coinsurance rate facing the family at that time. For example, if the insurance plan specifies a deductible, the effective coinsurance rate at the start of the year is 100 percent, and the occurrence of episodes is simulated assuming 100 percent coinsurance. As a family experiences episodes during the year, the effective coinsurance rate may change. For example, when the family's cumulative expenditures exceed the deductible, the effective coinsurance rate will fall to the nominal coinsurance rate specified in the plan. When the family's cumulative out-of-pocket maximum is reached, the effective coinsurance rate falls to zero for the rest of the year. The model keeps track of the total expenditures and family out-of-pocket expenditures throughout the year as episodes are generated. As the family's expenditures cause the effective coinsurance rate to change, the rate at which episodes are generated and the predicted expenditure of episodes that occur are adjusted accordingly.

Rather than directly adjust the Poisson rates to the effective coinsurance rate, the simulation model actually generates episodes for the family, assuming no cost sharing by the family, then randomly censors episodes if the individual remains responsible for a share of the cost. The episode loss rate at nonzero cost sharing is equal to one minus the observed HIE occurrence ratio for the effective cost sharing relative to that of no cost sharing. The cost of the episode is predicted assuming no cost sharing and adjusted downward in cost if the family is responsible for a share of the cost.

The procedure of censoring full-coverage episodes rather than changing the Poisson rates when the coinsurance rate changes has several advantages. First, it reduces the variance of the estimated difference in total expenditures between different insurance plans. Second, it allows us to realize catastrophic hospital episodes at the same rate irrespective of the effective coinsurance rates; that is, when the model predicts a catastrophic hospitalization, assuming full coverage, the hospitalization is not censored even if the effective coinsurance rate is greater than zero. This corresponds to the observation that when serious hospitalizations occurred, cost sharing had no effect. Third, it also allows us to realize more hospital episodes when families are close to their out-of-pocket limit than when the amount of out-of-pocket expenditures remaining is high. The HIE results indicated that when families are within about $1,125 (in 1989 dollars) of their out-of-pocket limit, they experience only about 10 percent fewer episodes than when the remaining out-of-pocket expenditure is higher (see Keeler et al., 1988, for a more complete description).

Using this simulation model, we can compute the effects on total health expenditures, insurance company payments, and out-of-pocket expenditures of different specifications of insurance coverage and cost sharing.

For this study, we simulated fee-for-service health-plan expenditures for a set of plans that looked like the current military health care benefit. The plan structure, that is, the copayment requirements, differed for active-duty families and retiree families. Within the active-duty population, the benefit was slightly more generous for enlisted families with rank up to E4. The plan structures for each of these groups are shown in Table E.5.

We estimated fee-for-service plan expenditures for three alternate samples: (1) the entire population, (2) individuals and families that selected a fee-for-service

136

Table E.5

**Current CHAMPUS Cost Sharing (used in simulating costs for
civilian fee-for-service plans)**

	Deductible	Inpatient and Cost Share	Outpatient and Cost Share	Cap
E1-E4	50	0	.20	1000
E5 and up	150	0	.20	1000
Retirees	150	.25	.25	7500

plan under alternative 3, and (3) individuals and families who selected a fee-for-service option under alternative 4. In all cases, we assumed that the active-duty members would obtain their health care through a separately arranged military health care option and thus eliminated them from our estimates.

Finally, for retirees we estimated an alternate fee-for-service health-plan benefit that looked like the Clinton health care plan.

Effects of Cost Sharing on Health Care Costs and Health Outcomes: The Health Insurance Experiment

The definitive study of the effects of cost sharing is the Health Insurance Experiment (HIE), conducted by RAND from 1974 through 1981. The experiment, which is documented in Newhouse (1994), enrolled 5,809 nonaged individuals randomly into 14 different fee-for-service insurance plans. The plans had different levels of cost sharing. The coinsurance rates tested were 0, 25, 50, and 95 percent, and the maximum levels of out-of-pocket expenditures were 5, 10, and 15 percent of family income (but no more than $1,000). The study followed these people for up to five years, collecting extensive data on their health care use, health status, and other outcomes related to health care.

The HIE data clearly show that the use of medical services responds to changes in the amount paid out of pocket. The per-capita expenses for health care on the free plan were 45 percent higher than on the plan with 95 percent coinsurance and 23 percent higher than on the 25 percent plan (coinsurance on all plans is subject to the limit on out-of-pocket costs of up to $1,000). Cost sharing primarily affects patient decisions to seek care, but has little effect on the amount of care delivered once care is initiated. Outpatient care is more responsive to cost sharing than inpatient care; in fact, inpatient care for children is unaffected by cost sharing. The response to cost sharing does not generally vary by income, health status, or local market characteristics. Cost sharing deterred contact with the medical system across the entire spectrum of illnesses and problems seen in the outpatient setting. However, the evidence does suggest that use of chronic care was less responsive than use of acute or preventive care. There was no difference in the rates of decrease according to the medical appropriateness of the service.

The study measured the effects of cost sharing on various measures of health:

- participants' ratings of their physical health, role functioning, mental health, social contacts, and general health;

- smoking behavior, weight, cholesterol level, diastolic blood pressure level, visual acuity, and an index of the risk of dying related to specific risk factors (systolic blood pressure, cholesterol, and smoking habits) in adults;

- anemia, hearing loss, fluid in the middle ear, and visual disorder in children.

Overall, the health effects measured were negligible. Free care did not affect the major health habits associated with cardiovascular disease and cancer in adults. It had at most a small effect on the general health measures for the average person. People having specific conditions with well-established diagnostic and therapeutic procedures (myopia, hypertension) benefited from free care, and these improvements appeared to be greater among the poor. It is possible that a longer follow-up of the participants would have uncovered health effects that were not apparent after three to five years. However, given the relatively high rates of inappropriate (i.e., potentially harmful) treatment documented in other studies, the researchers also concluded that, in the free plan, the positive effects of using more appropriate care may have been offset by the negative effects of using more inappropriate care.

Regression Models for Predicting MTF Utilization in Case 4

The methods used to estimate MTF utilization for case 4 were essentially the same as the methods used for cases 1 and 2. They are described in Appendices C and D. For case 4, we substituted the total visits and admissions for MTF visits and admissions in the regressions. We measured total utilization by summing military and civilian utilization reported in the beneficiary survey, substituting the self-reported civilian utilization data for CHAMPUS data because the former include utilization paid for by others. We assume that beneficiaries who would enroll in an MTF plan in case 4 would obtain all their care from that plan. Our health-plan choice models indicate that those with other insurance would generally enroll in civilian plans, where they could better coordinate their military and private coverage. We predicted utilization rates for case 4 using the same methods we used for case 2, with the exception that we did not expand the list of available MTFs beyond those operational in 1992. The regression models we estimated for case 4 are shown in Tables E.6–E.8.

Table E.6

Total Use for CHAMPUS-Eligible Adults in Catchment Areas

Variable	Probability of Visits>0		No. Visits if Visits>0		Probability: Hosp. Nights>0	
	Coefficient	Stand. Error	Coefficient	Stand. Error	Coefficient	Stand. Error
Intercept	-0.2334	0.2782	0.3028	0.1350	-1.2361	0.2814
Retired	-0.6941	0.1453	-0.1765	0.0651	-0.3741	0.1349
Retired female	0.3025	0.0585	0.1303	0.0248	-0.1910	0.0539
Officer	0.0970	0.0690	0.0275	0.0290	—	—
Not MTF service	-0.1615	0.0535	-0.0284	0.0233	-0.1390	0.0516
Employed	0.0007	0.0527	-0.0723	0.0233	-0.2935	0.0504
Family income	0.0685	0.0241	-0.0154	0.0098	-0.0727	0.0212
Family size	0.0291	0.0183	0.0217	0.0081	0.0601	0.0165
Age	0.0077	0.0121	0.0186	0.0056	0.0022	0.0119
Age squared	0.0000	0.0001	-0.0001	0.0001	0.0001	0.0001
Female age 18–34	0.2147	0.0818	0.2680	0.0395	0.2054	0.0824
No. health cond.	0.4254	0.0349	0.1685	0.0080	0.0834	0.0156
AFCAM enrolled	-0.4954	0.9379	0.0747	0.4323	-0.5209	0.3452
NAVCAM enrolled	1.4764	2.2675	-0.1079	0.2894	-0.4608	0.5003
CRI enrolled	0.7702	0.2144	0.1284	0.0677	0.0399	0.0978
AFCAM—ret.	-0.1908	0.9763	0.0221	0.4623	—	—
NAVCAM—ret.	-1.4925	2.3330	-0.1451	0.3827	—	—
CRI—ret.	-0.7533	0.2553	-0.0680	0.0912	—	—
Army MTF	0.1003	0.0584	0.0285	0.0246	-0.0129	0.0527
Navy MTF	-0.0255	0.0594	0.1277	0.0260	-0.0216	0.0556
log(MTF beds/pop.)	-0.1572	0.0851	0.0375	0.0361	0.0507	0.0776
log(beds/pop.)—ret.	0.1672	0.0967	0.0159	0.0415	0.0521	0.0889
log(MTF MDs/bed)	-0.0066	0.1535	0.1196	0.0617	0.1919	0.1324
log(MDs/bed)—ret.	0.2042	0.1788	-0.0063	0.0759	-0.3520	0.1617
Income—ret.	-0.0119	0.0252	0.0081	0.0101	0.0226	0.0237
Health cond.—ret.	0.0873	0.0423	-0.0215	0.0096	0.0504	0.0187
Privately insured	-0.1314	0.1189	-0.0679	0.0524	0.1118	0.1103
Priv. insured—ret.	0.4677	0.1323	0.2101	0.0584	0.0902	0.1239

Table E.7

Total Use for CHAMPUS-Eligible Children in Catchment Areas

Variable	Probability of Visits>0		No. Visits if Visits>0		Probability: Hosp. Nights>0	
	Coefficient	Stand. Error	Coefficient	Stand. Error	Coefficient	Stand. Error
Intercept	0.8520	0.1507	0.9899	0.0660	-0.0179	0.1572
Retired	0.2052	0.2456	0.1825	0.0956	0.0198	0.1651
Officer	0.3224	0.1147	-0.0770	0.0439	—	—
Not MTF service	-0.0638	0.0867	0.0597	0.0376	0.0965	0.0999
Employed	0.0406	0.0782	0.0229	0.0336	0.0697	0.0863
Family income	0.0350	0.0271	0.0232	0.0113	-0.0359	0.0220
Family size	-0.0258	0.0262	-0.0032	0.0114	-0.0145	0.0295
Age	-0.1294	0.0235	-0.0596	0.0099	-0.3920	0.0247
Age squared	0.0055	0.0014	0.0021	0.0006	0.0189	0.0015
No. health cond.	0.6826	0.0427	0.2910	0.0127	0.1139	0.0263
AFCAM enrolled	-0.3162	0.6296	0.0647	0.3027	0.9717	0.5039
NAVCAM enrolled	0.1396	0.7471	-0.0483	0.2888	0.4953	0.5553
CRI enrolled	0.0560	0.1331	-0.0800	0.0532	-0.0008	0.1266
AFCAM—ret.	4.9476	4444.0500	0.6258	0.5452	—	—
NAVYCAM—ret.	-0.7253	1.5040	0.5106	0.8531	—	—
CRI—ret.	-1.0083	0.3061	0.4185	0.1755		
Army MTF	-0.0733	0.0802	-0.0358	0.0339	0.0841	0.0895
Navy MTF	-0.0356	0.0869	0.0197	0.0359	0.1249	0.0946
log(MTF beds/pop.)	0.0011	0.0733	0.0134	0.0312	-0.0089	0.0784
log(MTF MDs/bed)	0.0044	0.1310	0.0728	0.0560	0.2789	0.1386
log(MDs/bed)—ret.	-0.0093	0.3033	0.3442	0.1164	0.0032	0.3414
log(beds/pop.)—ret.	-0.3215	0.1562	0.1415	0.0625	-0.0212	0.1843
Income—ret.	0.0293	0.0488	-0.0238	0.0160	—	—
Health cond.—ret.	-0.0485	0.0948	-0.0784	0.0233	—	—
Privately insured	-0.0909	0.1214	0.0133	0.0507	-0.0695	0.1302
Priv. insured—ret.	0.0402	0.2002	0.0973	0.0829	-0.4496	0.2504

Table E.8

Total Use for Medicare Eligibles in Catchment Areas

Variable	Probability of Visits>0		No. Visits if Visits>0		Probability: Hosp. Nights>0	
	Coefficient	Stand. Error	Coefficient	Stand. Error	Coefficient	Stand. Error
Intercept	1.1917	0.5017	1.2373	0.1841	-3.9396	0.3941
Officer	0.5930	0.1144	0.0002	0.0348	-0.5356	0.0784
Female	0.2311	0.0922	-0.0164	0.0306	0.1195	0.0659
Not MTF service	-0.1961	0.0860	-0.0162	0.0292	-0.1561	0.0642
Family income	-0.0587	0.0236	0.0613	0.0078	0.0916	0.0165
Family size	-0.5370	0.0991	-0.1261	0.0354	-0.0659	0.0771
Age	-0.0079	0.0071	-0.0031	0.0025	0.0398	0.0054
No. health cond.	0.2747	0.0276	0.1361	0.0058	0.1197	0.0123
Army MTF	0.5056	0.1046	-0.0804	0.0349	-0.3574	0.0759
Navy MTF	0.2381	0.1038	-0.1801	0.0366	-0.1820	0.0781
log(MTF beds/pop.)	-0.2584	0.0782	0.0332	0.0260	0.0190	0.0566
log(MTF MDs/bed)	-0.2162	0.1566	0.0712	0.0511	0.0272	0.1109

F. SURVEY QUESTIONS USED TO PREDICT HEALTH PLAN CHOICE

SUPPOSE THERE WAS A <u>NEW KIND OF MILITARY HEALTH PLAN</u> AND YOU COULD CHOOSE THE NEW PLAN OR CONTINUE TO GET YOUR HEALTH CARE THE WAY YOU DO NOW. QUESTIONS 105 AND 106 ASK YOU TO COMPARE YOUR <u>CURRENT MILITARY PLAN</u> AS IT IS NOW WITH TWO NEW PLANS, AND TO ANSWER WHETHER OR NOT YOU WOULD CHANGE.

> IMPORTANT: ANSWERING THESE QUESTIONS <u>WILL NOT</u> AFFECT YOUR CURRENT MILITARY HEALTH PLAN. THESE QUESTIONS ARE FOR RESEARCH PURPOSES ONLY AND DO NOT DESCRIBE ACTUAL PLANS THAT EXIST NOW.

105. The first new military health plan we want you to consider is a CIVILIAN Health Maintenance Organization or HMO. Suppose this plan offered the services and benefits listed in Table 1 below. A decision to change to this plan means you would use it instead of Military Medical Treatment Facilities or CHAMPUS.

TABLE 1: DESCRIPTION OF NEW MILITARY HEALTH PLAN #1

SERVICES COVERED:	Same as CHAMPUS but includes adult annual physical exams and routine eye care.
CHOOSING YOUR HOSPITAL AND DOCTOR	
CHOOSING A HOSPITAL:	Use the civilian hospital associated with the plan.
CHOOSING A DOCTOR:	Visit any doctor at the plan facility.
YOUR SHARE OF THE COST OF SERVICES	
HOSPITAL STAYS:	No charge for sponsor or family members.
OUTPATIENT DOCTOR VISITS:	Sponsor and family members pay $5 per visit.
YOUR ABILITY TO GET AN APPOINTMENT:	For routine physical exam: appointment in 3 days. For illness that is not serious: appointment in 2 days. For serious illness: same day appointment. If care is not available from the plan's doctor, you will be sent to another doctor.

Would you join this new plan instead of your current MILITARY HEALTH PLAN?

	Yes	No
a. If there was a charge of $75 per month per family	O	O
b. If there was a charge of $50 per month per family	O	O
c. If there was no charge to join	O	O

106. The second new military health plan we want you to consider is a military HMO. This plan would offer the benefits and services listed in Table 2 below. A decision to change to this plan means you would no longer be able to use CHAMPUS. If you do not live near a military hospital, consider what you would prefer if you did live near a military hospital.

TABLE 2: DESCRIPTION OF NEW MILITARY HEALTH PLAN #2

SERVICES COVERED:	Same as CHAMPUS but includes adult annual physical exams and routine eye care.
CHOOSING YOUR HOSPITAL AND DOCTOR	
CHOOSING A HOSPITAL:	Use the military hospital.
CHOOSING A DOCTOR:	Visit doctor at the military hospital.
YOUR SHARE OF THE COST OF SERVICES	
HOSPITAL STAYS:	No charge for sponsor or family members.
OUTPATIENT DOCTOR VISITS:	Sponsor and family members pay $5 per visit.
YOUR ABILITY TO GET AN APPOINTMENT:	For routine physical exam: appointment in 3 days. For illness that is not serious: appointment in 2 days. For serious illness: same day appointment. If care is not available from the plan's doctor, you will be sent to another doctor.

Would you join this new plan instead of your current MILITARY HEALTH PLAN?

	Yes	No
a. If there was a charge of $75 per month per family	O	O
b. If there was a charge of $50 per month per family	O	O
c. If there was no charge to join	O	O

References

Amemiya, T., *Advanced Econometrics*, Cambridge, Mass: Harvard University Press, 1985.

Bradbury, Robert C., Joseph H. Golec, and Frank E. Stearns, "Comparing Hospital Length of Stay in Independent Practice Association HMOs and Traditional Insurance Programs," *Inquiry*, Vol. 28, Spring 1991, pp. 87–93.

Brook, Robert H., et al., *The Effect of Coinsurance on the Health of Adults: Results from the RAND Health Insurance Experiment*, Santa Monica, Calif.: RAND, R-3055-HHS, 1984.

Buchanan, Joan L., et al., "Simulating Health Expenditures Under Alternative Insurance Plans," *Management Science*, Vol. 37, No. 7, 1991, pp. 1067–1090.

Congressional Budget Office, *An Analysis of the Administration's Health Proposal*, Washington, D.C., February 1994.

Congressional Budget Office, *Evaluating the Costs of Expanding the CHAMPUS Reform Initiative into Washington and Oregon*, Washington, D.C., November 1993.

Congressional Budget Office, *Reforming the Military Health Care System*, Washington, D.C., January 1988.

Department of Defense, *The Economics of Sizing the Military Medical Establishment: Executive Report of the Comprehensive Study of the Military Medical Care System*, April 1994.

Duan, Naihua, "Smearing Estimate: A Nonparametric Retransformation Method," *Journal of the American Statistical Association*, Vol. 78, No. 383, September 1983, pp. 605–610.

Duan, Naihua, et al., *A Comparison of Alternative Models for the Demand for Medical Care*, Santa Monica, Calif.: RAND, R-2754-HHS, 1982.

Garnick, Deborah W., et al., "Services and Charges by PPO Physicians for PPO and Indemnity Patients: An Episode of Care Comparison," *Medical Care*, Vol. 28, No. 10, October 1990, pp. 894–917.

Goldberg, Matthew, et al., *Cost Analysis of the Military Medical Care System: Final Report*, Alexandria, Va.: Institute for Defense Analyses, P-2990, September 1994.

Hosek, Susan D., Dana P. Goldman, Lloyd S. Dixon, and Elizabeth S. Sloss, *Evaluation of the CHAMPUS Reform Initiative: Vol. 3, Health Care Utilization and Costs*, Santa Monica, Calif.: RAND, R-4244/3-HA, 1993.

Huber, P. J., "The Behavior of Maximum Likelihood Estimates Under Nonstandard Conditions," *Fifth Berkeley Symposium of Mathematical Statistics and Probability*, Vol. 1, 1967, pp. 221–233.

Jobe, Jaren B., Andrew A. White, Catherine L. Kelley, David J. Mingay, Marcus J. Sanchez, and Elizabeth F. Loftus, "Recall Strategies and Memory for Health-Care Visits," *The Milbank Quarterly*, Vol. 68, No. 2, 1990.

Keeler, Emmett B., et al., "Hospital Characteristics and Quality of Care," *JAMA*, October 7, 1992, pp. 1709–1714.

Keeler, Emmett B., et al., *The Demand for Episodes of Medical Treatment in the Health Insurance Experiment*, Santa Monica, Calif.: RAND, R-3454-HHS, 1988.

Kennell, David, Terry Savela, Ron Mitchell, and Charles Roehrig, "Report on the PRIMUS/NAVCARE Programs," unpublished report to the Department of Defense, Lewin/ICF and Vector Research, Inc., May 1991.

Kronick, Richard, David C. Goodman, John Wennberg, and Edward Wagner, "The Marketplace in Health Care Reform," *The New England Journal of Medicine*, January 14, 1993, pp. 149–150.

Lewin-VHI, Inc., "Overview of Lewin-VHI Certification Analysis Assumptions," unpublished report to the Department of Defense, February 1993a.

Lewin-VHI, Inc., "Revised Estimates of Competitive Effects and Structural Improvements," unpublished memorandum to the Department of Defense, August 1993b.

Luft, Harold S., *Health Maintenance Organizations: Dimensions of Performance*, New York: John Wiley, 1981.

Luft, Harold S., "The Relation between Surgical Volume and Mortality: An Exploration of Casual Factors and Alternative Models," *Medical Care*, September 1980, pp. 940–959.

Luft, Harold S., et al., "Should Operations Be Regionalized? The Empirical Relation Between Surgical Volume and Mortality," *The New England Journal of Medicine*, December 20, 1979, pp. 1364–1369.

Lurie, Phillip M., Karen W. Tyson, Michael L. Fineberg, Larry A. Waisanen, James A. Roberts, Mark E. Sieffert, and Bette S. Mahoney, *Analysis of the 1992 DoD Survey of Military Medical Care Beneficiaries*, Alexandria, Va.: Institute for Defense Analyses, 1994.

Manning, W. G., and M. S. Marquis, *Health Insurance: The Trade-Off Between Risk Pooling and Moral Hazard*, Santa Monica, Calif.: RAND, R-3729-NCHSR, 1989.

Manning, Willard G., et al., "A Controlled Trial of the Effect of a Prepaid Group Practice on Use of Service," *New England Journal of Medicine*, Vol. 310, 1984, pp. 1505–1510.

Marquis, M. S., D. E. Kanouse, L. Brodsley, *Informing Consumers About Health Care Costs: A Review and Research Agenda*, Santa Monica, Calif.: RAND, R-3262-HCFA, 1985.

National Center for Health Statistics, "Current Estimates from the National Health Interview Survey, 1989," *Vital Health Statistics*, Vol. 10, No. 176, 1990.

Newhouse, Joseph P., et al., *Free for All? Lessons from the RAND Health Insurance Experiment*, Cambridge, Mass: Harvard University Press, 1994.

Phelps, Charles E., Susan D. Hosek, Joan L. Buchanan, Adele R. Palmer, Kathleen N. Lohr, and Christina Witsberger, *Health Care in the Military: Feasibility and Desirability of a Health Enrollment System*, Santa Monica, Calif.: RAND, R-3145-HA, 1984.

Siemiatycki, Jack, "A Comparison of Mail, Telephone, and Home Interview Strategies for Household Health Surveys," *AJPH*, Vol. 69, No. 3, March, 1979, pp. 238–245.

Sloss, Elizabeth M., and Susan D. Hosek, *Evaluation of the CHAMPUS Reform Initiative: Vol. 2, Beneficiary Access and Satisfaction*, Santa Monica, Calif.: RAND, R-4244/2-HA, 1993.

U.S. Department of Health and Human Services, Social Security Administration, *Annual Statistical Supplement, 1993 to the Social Security Bulletin*, Washington, D.C., August 1993.

Welch, W. P., "Health Care Utilization in HMO's: Results from Two National Samples," *Journal of Health Economics*, No. 4, December 1985, pp. 293–308.

Wouters, Annemarie V., "The Cost of Acute Outpatient Primary Care in Preferred Provider Organization," *Medical Care*, Vol. 28, No. 7, July 1990, pp. 573–585.